D0359574

I Feel You

I Feel You

The Surprising Power
of Extreme Empathy

CRIS BEAM

An Eamon Dolan Book

HOUGHTON MIFFLIN HARCOURT

BOSTON   NEW YORK

2018

For information about permission to reproduce selections from this book,
write to trade.permissions@hmhco.com or to Permissions,
Houghton Mifflin Harcourt Publishing Company,
3 Park Avenue, 19th Floor, New York, New York 10016.

hmhco.com

Library of Congress Cataloging-in-Publication Data
Names: Beam, Cris, author.
Title: I feel you : the surprising power of extreme empathy / Cris Beam.
Description: Boston : Houghton Mifflin Harcourt, 2018. |
Includes bibliographical references and index.
Identifiers: LCCN 2017045815 (print) | LCCN 2017052085 (ebook) |
ISBN 9780544558175 (ebook) | ISBN 9780544558168 (hardback)
Subjects: LCSH: Empathy. | Emotions. | BISAC: PSYCHOLOGY / Emotions. |
PSYCHOLOGY / Interpersonal Relations. | PSYCHOLOGY / General.
Classification: LCC BF575.E55 (ebook) | LCC BF575.E55 B43 2018 (print) |
DDC 152.4/1 — dc23
LC record available at https://lccn.loc.gov/2017045815

Book design by Victoria Hartman

Printed in the United States of America
DOC 10 9 8 7 6 5 4 3 2 1

Excerpt from "Islands" (1976) by Muriel Rukeyser
used by permission of the estate of Muriel Rukeyser.

FOR TERESA

ISLANDS

O for God's sake
they are connected
underneath . . .

— MURIEL RUKEYSER

Contents

Author's Note

This is a work of nonfiction. A very few names have been changed to protect identities; these are marked in the text or in notes at the back of the book.

Introduction

Every generation, a phrase enters the American consciousness and interrupts collective action like a boulder changing the course of a stream. In the 1960s, the phrase was civil rights; in the 1980s, it was self-esteem; now our word is empathy. Like the terms that came before it, empathy sounds redemptive—it's an orientation that, should we adopt it en masse, could extricate us from our violence and our greed. But it's also a term so varied in meaning and slippery in application, it can have ambiguous, even deleterious, effects. Empathy, when applied artfully and in the right contexts, can be highly moral and deeply liberating—but it's not an empty gesture to be spread atop every interaction in this new and troubled millennium. We have to understand both its purpose and practice, and this book is an attempt to do just that.

One example that can stand in for many: In the aftermath of the 2016 election, empathy has been weaponized. On one side, progressives argue that an empathy deficit, in part, is to blame for how the election blindsided them; when they thought Hillary Clinton was a shoo-in, a paucity of imagination kept them from truly seeing the swath of voters that could choose Donald Trump. Now many on the left feel they need to deploy empathy, in a gesture of unity and understanding that was so clearly missing in 2016. On the other side, voices have erupted in a chorus *against* empathy for Trump supporters: Trump is a bigot, they cry, and if he (and they) can't have empathy for us, why should we have empathy for them?

But I have learned in writing this book that empathy is not one singular thing. It can, when it's contextualized the way it is above, serve as a way to be meek and deferential, or as a tool to withhold from political enemies, but it can also be instead an immediate gesture of common humanity. It can be innate, elemental, as difficult to stanch as love. Other times, empathy operates as a kind of karmic loop: empathy for the one affects the whole and vice versa. So what are we talking about when we talk about empathy?

One arena that's directing our current American associations with the word is the corporate one, so let's start with the place many of us begin our days: on Facebook. For years, Facebook users pressured headquarters to create a "dislike" button, but Mark Zuckerberg wouldn't bite. He admitted that some posts are sad or maddening or anything but "likable" but said disliking wasn't the online culture he wanted to build. Instead, in 2015, he said he planned to incorporate some kind of clickable empathy button. Facebook came out with four emoji faces: happy, sad, surprised, and angry—new emblems to say, "I see your post, and I feel your pain."

Mark Zuckerberg may hope his 1.5 billion monthly users feel like they're feeling more—but the richer our experience, the richer Facebook becomes. Online, we are both the consumer and the product, as Facebook earns $5.84 billion a quarter selling our demographics and our likes. In these days of DVR and streaming, corporations can no longer rely on the mass-market commercial to reach an audience; instead they count on courting us individually online. When we buy dog food one day and find a charticle from Purina in our newsfeed the next, we no longer find it strange—we know our electronic DNA is scattered on every screen we touch to be gathered and sold to marketers. Some may find this comforting, and some may call it surveillance, but what's interesting is what the corporations call it: empathy.

Empathic marketing, empathic branding—these are the hot corporate buzzwords wending their way through business schools and ad agencies now. "Corporate Empathy Is Not an Oxymoron." So reads a recent *Harvard Business Review* headline, with the claim that "enlightened companies are increasingly aware that delivering empathy for their customers, employees, and the public is a powerful tool for improving profits."

This corporate definition of empathy connotes getting to know and understand a consumer base—our tastes, our spending habits, our personal needs—to sell us more stuff. "Empathic design" is another burgeoning field, wherein marketers and designers work with people to identify latent needs and feelings about certain products and then, from that information, build new things to sell them.

You could argue that the corporate world's commodification of empathy is simply the bastardization of a term, but I'd argue that something deeper is afoot. Capitalism is milking the trend of all things empathy, but it's also building a culture that perverts our very understanding of the concept. In other words, as we expect our watches, our phones, our computers, to provide us with experiences curated solely for us, we feel *empathized with* in a particular way, which has led consumers to need a particular kind of empathy. Through our everyday interactions with commerce, we attune to a cultural value shift that marks empathy as acquisitional and profitable.

For example, in education: In a recent *Education Week* article, the author defines empathy as a skill and advises teachers to create lesson plans in empathic design. Another, titled "Empathy, Strategy and Edupreneurship: Fostering a Culture of Innovation," cites increased student learning as the "profit" of the classroom. In one *Forbes* article, called "Why We Should Teach Empathy to Improve Education (and Test Scores)," the writer comes from Ashoka, the $70 million nonprofit founded by management consultant Bill Drayton to support social entrepreneurs across the globe. This is an instance of Ashoka's content marketing in mainstream journalism. One of Ashoka's projects is called the "Empathy Initiative," whose goal is "to create a world committed and equipped to ensuring that every child masters empathy." I'm fascinated by this messianic notion, and when I interviewed Ashoka's director, by her assertion that "we live in a world that values success *and* values empathy. Companies are clamoring for this skill."

In this book, I cast a critical gaze on both this impetus for empathy and the type of empathy we're clamoring for — as empathy, the movement, continues to gain ground. After all, at first blush, empathy sounds perfectly desirable. It sounds like it's about understanding and even caring for your fellow human beings, a precursor to a fair society. But I worry about the ways empathy is increasingly positioned as a skill, something to be coveted and calculated, rather than a more ineffable ethic or a value, practiced out of instinct and for some intrinsic moral good. So in *I Feel You,* I've looked to the places outside of this paradigm: to the places we're seeing empathy applied, right now, in creative, unusual, and ultimately useful ways.

I've divided the book into three parts. In part 1, Understanding, I break down the various ways we both understand empathy as a concept and *use* empathy to understand the other, one to one. I begin *I Feel You* in the neuroscience labs of Southern California, where researchers study mirror neurons, sometimes called empathy neurons or even Gandhi neurons, and whose discovery is credited with launching the empathy avalanche. From there, I explore the landscape of elementary schools, where innovators are teaching children about empathy in surprising ways — and where a debate rages over what empathy actually is. Some say empathy is a skill and should be taught that way, while others claim it's a moral inclination. I myself take a class on empathic listening for adults and try to apply the tools. I also spend some time thinking about artistic empathy, with a performance artist and a youth storytelling group with a fervent mission to spread empathy across the globe.

All of this leads me to think about what empathy is *for*, and part 2, Justice, is about moving empathy into action. Outside of the corporate sphere, there's a prosocial element to the idea of empathy — an antecedent to getting along, to good citizenship, or to justice. To understand the idea of empathy and justice, I looked at two courts: one a restitutional justice program and the other, the new Human Trafficking Intervention Court (HTIC) in New York. The HTIC launched in 2013 with the idea that people arrested for prostitution should no longer be prosecuted as criminals but rather be seen as victims and offered social services instead.

From there I go to Maine, where the idea of empathy and justice has moved out of the courts entirely. This is part 3 of the book: Forgiveness. For the past few years, the state of Maine and the five Wabanaki tribes have been conducting a Truth and Reconciliation Commission (TRC), modeled loosely after the TRC in South Africa. Here, empathy shifts out of the empathy-as-helping model and into empathy as bearing witness. In Maine, some felt the purpose of engendering empathy for one's former adversary was to foster forgiveness; others asked how forgiveness could truly be offered when each participant in this exchange was treading on the bones of a five-hundred-year history of colonialism. In other words, when people use the naive expression "standing in another's shoes," they must think not only of the shoes but also the ground underneath.

One person who addresses this need for empathic exchanges informed by context and history is Pumla Gobodo-Madikizela, a nationally recognized South African psychoanalyst who served on the original TRC and, when I met her, ran an institute called Trauma, Forgiveness, and Reconciliation Studies at the University of the Free State in Bloemfontein. Her current research is on the development of empathy in victim-perpetrator dialogue in the aftermath of mass violence and genocide. I spent three weeks with Gobodo-Madikizela in South Africa, where, in part 3, I explore what it means to use empathy to forgive an impossible other, a genocidal state, an enemy. I look to the most difficult empathy of all, both intimate and faceless: those who have committed gross violations against us. I explore my own past and family relationships fraught with violence and neglect, and I meet with those who have faced down murderers of their loved ones and found a common humanity. In South Africa, it's the second generation that's now explicitly navigating their way through a public empathy between groups that have historically learned to objectify one another. This navigation is particularly present at the universities, like the one where Gobodo-Madikizela teaches and where I interviewed dozens of students who claimed reconciliation as an ongoing social demand. Students, by and large, have eschewed the notion of the "big violators" of their parents' generation and adopted instead the idea that inside each of them is the "little perpetrator," who must always be challenged in kind and empathic public dialogue, lest apartheid rise again. I found these dialogues both totally unfamiliar and potentially very useful for other contexts. In this way, *I Feel You* is a journey both critical and creative, juxtaposing analysis of our current empathy overload with a narrative exploration of many empathic experiments that can be applied to the equally stratified and ruptured times in which we live.

· PART I ·

Understanding

1

The Sound of Science

In the Arkansas town of Conway, tens of thousands of computer servers churn together day and night, swallowing up our secrets. They belong to a giant corporation called Acxiom, a data broker that pulls in more than $800 million a year by culling information about people's online behaviors and demographics, typecasting us all into elderly singles or Subaru-driving cat lovers, and then selling that intel to marketers across the globe. While I believe this growing capitalist trend of targeting each consumer individually, of mirroring our habits with products more and more precisely, is the real fuel behind America's drive toward all things empathy, it doesn't make a very pretty story.

So we tell a different one. We tell a story about a monkey lab in Parma, Italy, and the way those monkeys led us to change everything we thought we knew about empathy.

Giacomo Rizzolatti looks something like Albert Einstein, with the same mane of white hair, a similar bushy mustache, and when he talks in public it's with a genuine smile in his voice. Rizzolatti directs the lab that discovered mirror neurons in the motor cortex of macaque monkeys. Mirror neurons, unlike other neurons in the motor region that fire when the monkey moves, instead also fire when the monkey simply *watches someone else* performing a motor task. When they first found these neurons some fifteen years ago, Rizzolatti and his team thought they must have been making a mistake: motor neurons only fired to direct bodily movement, they believed, so the monkey was probably moving somehow — maybe a pinkie finger twitch — without their detection. When they repeated the test and realized these neurons fired simply in response to *witnessing* motorization in somebody else, they had a major publication on their hands.

Nature rejected their paper. Only physiologists, the editors claimed, would be interested in this discovery — which was too narrow for their broad readership. So the team went elsewhere, publishing in a more specialized journal, and the idea blasted outside its borders: the paper has been cited thousands of times and launched incalculable studies in multiple fields. As Rizzolatti said, this happened because one very famous scientist — the charismatic man who developed therapy for patients with phantom limb pain and who writes popular books about people who taste colors, experience psychological pregnancies, and other neurological oddities — was to name Rizzolatti's mirror neuron study the most important paper published in the ten years prior to 2000. The man was V. S. Ramachandran.

When this happened, Rizzolatti said, "it was a tremendous boost . . . A lot of people outside physiology — sociologists, philosophers, psychologists, others — said, 'Perhaps we have found a mechanism that can explain many things.'"

The mechanism was the proof, the neurological seedling that could grow into one very human narrative of empathy. *Monkey see, monkey do* had earned an extra step: monkey sees you do and feels it too. A neuron coded for reflecting movement without moving a muscle was freighted with meaning. Primates (and, by extension, humans) could actually *experience the other inside their own brains.* With the Parma discovery, empathy wasn't a utopian wish, or a socially constructed behavior: it was a neurological fact. And this was the story that made empathy come alive.

. . .

BEFORE ANY ITALIAN MACAQUES were bolted to their primate chairs to watch men pick up peanuts again and again, there was one predominantly accepted understanding of empathic learning. It went like this: a person (say, a child) has one expectation about the outside world, based on his past experience. The child forms a theory—when Mommy cries, it means she's sad. When one day Mommy cries from joy, the child revises his theory: another's tears can indicate sadness *or* happiness. Through increasingly complex experiences, we keep building increasingly complex theories about others' states of mind, their motivations, and so on. This is called theory-theory.

In the macaque's brains, experimenters didn't see theory-theory happening—they saw something much more basic and self-centered. Monkeys' *grasping* neurons fired when they witnessed someone merely *reaching* toward an apple. They were understanding the other's state of mind (wanting to pick up an apple) by mentalizing the action themselves. In a famous paper, philosophy and cognitive science professor Alvin Goldman teamed up with Vittorio Gallese from the Parma team to suggest that mirror neurons "underlie the process of 'mind-reading,'" or serve as precursors to such a process.

Mind-reading isn't as mystical as it sounds. It's simply, as Goldman and Gallese describe in their paper, the "activity of representing specific mental states of others, for example, their perceptions, goals, beliefs, expectations, and the like." It's pretty much accepted that children are adept at mind-reading by the age of four—when they start to lie.

Before the discovery of mirror neurons, in other words, everybody knew that we could all project ourselves into other people's perspectives: we just didn't know *how*. Neuroscientists had placed their bets on the theory-theory; others proposed what's called the simulation theory, which posited that our cognition of others' experiences came from somehow replicating their actions or states internally. Mirror neurons unequivocally favored this approach.

This idea became the cornerstone of the enormous buildup of all things empathy. Psychologists, neuroscientists, businesspeople, laypeople, had found their holy grail: mirror neurons supposedly revealed how we took on the perspective of another—we simulated it, we felt it, directly in our brains. Everybody, it seemed, took up the cause, and this remains one major conceptualization of empathy today.

This multidisciplinary surge to find meaning in empathy seems to run in cycles. Every hundred years or so, whenever current intellectual trends tend to champion rational thought and individualism, someone comes up with a new definition or mechanism for empathy.

A little under two hundred years ago, before the word "empathy" had been coined, David Hume and Adam Smith wrote extensively about "sympathy." That word didn't have the same pitying undertones it carries now; it denoted an eighteenth-century definition of sympathy wherein Hume wrote about mirroring as an essential human trait, and Smith said that it went further, claiming that sympathizing required both imagination and understanding the context from which another's emotion comes.

Hume and Smith were responding in part to the egoist philosophy of the day, promoted by people like Thomas Hobbes and Jean-Jacques Rousseau, with his "savage" man. The egoists claimed that men will act, first and foremost, in their own self-interest. Hume called this the "selfish hypothesis." He looked for evidence that we're more than mercenary, greedy beasts. For a while, newly celebrated sympathy found its way into all kinds of disciplines: physicians used the term to describe communication between organs, and the 1797 *Encyclopedia Britannica* had an entry for "somatic sympathy." Novels shifted toward the sentimental—with all their swooning, tears, and melancholia, and readers loved the books for the sympathies they evoked.

Soon enough, however, the novels were mocked for their hysteria, and physicians were looking for more precise, less occult-sounding terminology. Sympathy fell out of favor.

By the end of the nineteenth century, the pendulum had swung back toward another "selfish hypothesis" with Friedrich Nietzsche's ideas of the superman and his revolutionary belief that the only intentional part of human nature is the will to power. In art, abstract formalism ruled: artists and their admirers talked of the aesthetic appeal of shapes and proportions, and sought to develop a "science of forms." But adherents to the Romantic Movement rebelled — they knew that art evoked feelings and that feelings mattered — and this was the fertile soil in which empathy again could bloom.

Empathy, the word, is barely a hundred years old, and it began in fact as an aesthetic concept. It was first written as *Einfühlung*, which means "feeling into." That term was coined by a philosopher named Robert Vischer but popularized by another German philosopher, Theodor Lipps, who wrote dense, scholarly treatises on the supposed natural, inherent instinct humans have to translate aesthetic experiences into bodily ones. It works like this: say you're looking at a Doric column. You don't simply take in the dimensions of the column with your eyes, but you *feel* it with your body. Without literally moving, you'll sense yourself as the Doric column, experiencing a straightening.

Lipps described this experience as quick, perhaps even unconscious, a notion that would later influence Sigmund Freud. *Einfühlung,* the idea that we instantaneously and unintentionally project ourselves into objects — and, as Lipps later theorized, into other people — was controversial but astonishingly far-reaching. By the beginning of the twentieth century (much like the beginning of the twenty-first), empathy was a force to be reckoned with, wending its way into a range of disciplines — aesthetics, of course, but also psychology, hermeneutics, and phenomenology. As part of the swing away from the rational and toward the experiential, numerous thinkers took up this concept of "feeling into" another. They recognized it intuitively as a lived experience but did battle over its precise purpose and application. Phenomenologists, for instance, were interested in empathy as a form of consciousness, but they took issue with Lipps's insistence on fusion, as it presumes the "other" is the same as "me." Empathy is more useful, they thought, as a way to directly experience another's emotions, but it serves another function too: empathy allows us to experience ways others understand us.

And now here we are again. Just before mirror neurons were discovered, Western philosophers had been mired in poststructuralism and postmodernism — battle cries against mushy universals and feel-good humanism. I came of age when postmodernism cast its hue over most humanities, and I still find its precepts freeing. But all that careful scrutiny of power and social constructions, all the identity politics of the 1980s and 1990s that made way for the more shifting or fluid identities of the 1990s and 2000s, can create a longing for something fixed and inherent. The cult of increasingly specialized and curated personal identities (as opposed to national identities, religious identities, and so on), and the glut of selfies showcased on social media, seem to be the "selfish hypothesis" of our day. And yet we're shifting: French philosophers like Michel Foucault urged us into our identity politics; now contemporary pop philosophers like Alain de Botton command us to unplug from our Twitter podiums to tune in to deeper feelings. The pendulum is swinging back toward feeling, back toward love and the communal. Back toward empathy.

AFTER THE PARMA GROUP documented the mirror neurons' existence, neuroscientists all over the world began looking for them in humans, using technologies like functional magnetic resonance imaging and transcranial magnetic stimulation and a host of other systems that capture the brain's activity in general regions, rather than isolated points. Rizzolatti kept going with his monkeys, and these multiple groups started seeing the exact same thing: humans, like the macaques, possess mirror neurons in the motor cortex. When we observe someone else grasping that apple, a subset of our motor neurons will fire as though we were grasping it too. Humans, like monkeys, don't just process another's actions visually; we "act it out" in the brain, without moving a muscle.

And then, apparently, we extrapolate. TED Talks are good places for this. In a 2009 presentation cinematically titled "Neurons That Shaped Civilization," V. S. Ramachandran, the popular neuroscientist, launched mirror neurons into the limelight. He said he liked to call mirror neurons "empathy neurons." Ramachandran described research that had emerged since the Parma discovery, claiming that mirror neurons definitely existed in humans, particularly in the sensory processing regions. In reality, because we can't pry open human skulls and pop in electrodes, only songbirds had been added to the certifiable mirror neuron list—and only in the motor region. But fMRI studies in the Netherlands indicated that certain parts of the brain lit up when a person watched someone else being touched—and many scientists, including Ramachandran, made the leap. "We have mirror neurons for touch," he said, and he personified them. "It's as though the motor neurons are adopting the other person's point of view."

Ramachandran has since been taken to task for many of his claims—including his supposition that a sudden emergence of a sophisticated mirror neuron system some fifty thousand years ago spawned the great leap forward, when Homo sapiens began using tools and making art. But still, as TED Talks critics have often observed, complicated science was burned down to a bright ember and people left with the smoke it emitted. Ramachandran claimed mirror neurons make us "empathize" with another person being touched, but touch and pain receptors in our skin form a "feedback loop" into our own brains, letting us know it is not our own skin feeling the squeeze. Ramachandran said simple anesthesia would allow you to feel the vision of another person being pinched or squeezed as your own pain. "Remove the skin and you experience that person's touch in your mind. You've removed the barrier between you and other human beings," he said. And herein lies the smoke. "There is no real distinction between your consciousness and somebody else's consciousness. This is not just some mumbo-jumbo philosophy. This emerges from our basic understanding of neuroscience."

Back when Rizzolatti made his discovery, he was surprised by the range of people in the range of disciplines that showed an interest in his mirror neurons: they were, after all, in a discrete brain region in one particular animal. The psychologists, especially, he said, found it "a bit hard to accept that it was in the motor system because they always considered the motor system something rather dull and stupid."

This turned out not to matter. In 2000, Ramachandran predicted that mirror neurons would do for psychology what DNA had done for biology. Neuroscientists brought the idea of mirror neurons right to psychology's front door.

Despite the fact that we haven't seen them in humans, not in the same way we've seen them in monkeys, mirror neurons have been linked to (among other things) mass hysteria, contagious yawning, obesity, stuttering, business leadership, and the misattribution of anger in music. The backlash against such spurious connections of late has been bright and fierce.

Maybe it's too easy for me to say, as a non-scientist looking in through a window at wires and monkeys and imaging machines, that in the rush to denounce shaky science, we might be missing a key point: the spillage. When a discovery is so promising in its potential, or so poetic in its resonance with lived experience, then it spills out of its laboratory confines. Scientists and non-scientists both use the core concept as a generative spark for more experiments: it becomes an idea available to anyone, anywhere, to germinate and grow.

· · ·

PRIMATE LABS ARE NOT the most empathic places, at least from the monkeys' perspective. The scientists in Parma complied with the European law on the humane care and use of lab animals, which meant that they could anesthetize two macaques, remove part of the bone from the skull, and cement a small chamber to the hole, through which they would later insert their micro-electrodes. They also cemented a device to the bone that would hold the monkey's head completely still while she sat in her primate chair for her experiments.

As the brain itself has no pain receptors, the two monkeys couldn't feel the tungsten electrodes, which look like long, thin needles, passing through their dura and into their cortex. Rizzolatti's team was looking to isolate individual neurons in the premotor region called the F5. Rizzolatti had already spent a lot of time in this area, with other monkeys. He helped establish a map of its complex visual, motor, and tactile fields. When the Parma team began their experiments on the two macaques, they knew the neurons in the F5 region correlated to hand and mouth movements, and that the hand-related neurons discharged selectively — during goal-related motions like grasping or manipulating. And they knew that certain neurons were coded for specific kinds of hand prehension like a precision grip, and that others only fired in the presence of a 3-D object or if there was a match between that object's size and the type of grasp it required. In other words, this was a region that transformed visual information about an object into the potential for picking it up.

Macaque brains are only about a quarter of the size of the average human's, and they have a much smaller neocortex. That's the most recently evolved region, and in people it controls higher functions like language, reasoning, and conscious thought. Macaques present some social parallels to humans — notably, the mothers bond with their infants — but they're also different. For example, they organize themselves along matrilineal lines wherein the youngest daughter outranks her older sisters. Biologically, they're not as close to us as the bonobo or the chimpanzee—with whom we share 99 percent of our DNA. Rizzolatti was limited to studying macaques because European ethics regulations don't allow for experimenting on the great apes who, like humans, often walk upright, create tools and beds, communicate with language, manipulate one another with rage and sex, and can learn to use computers. In the Balearic Islands, Spain, great apes have been granted legal personhood, and there have been arguments to reclassify them in the *Homo* genus grouping, like us. All of this to say that there's a philosophy behind the philosophy: certain animals are marked as closer to the top of the species tree and thus endowed with more rights to evade medical study and suffering. We have the most empathy for animals most similar to us. Still, when scientists pluck subjects from farther down the tree, do the parallels falter?

I find it ironic that, while we may not exactly abuse animals in our search for human empathy, we certainly disturb them quite a bit. Sixty years ago, researchers were outright inhumane to rhesus macaques in one ongoing study—yet it also influenced thinkers in multiple fields. This older study bears out other parallels too, particularly in the way the language *about* a discovery influences the outcroppings from the discovery itself.

These days, scientists know enough to hide the actual sight of monkey suffering behind the jargon of academic journals, but back in the 1950s, camera crews filmed a fledgling colony of monkeys housed in a formerly vacant building down the street from the University of Wisconsin–Madison. The lab director, Harry Harlow, was proud of his results: orphaned baby monkeys who preferred simulated cloth mothers over wire monkeys that dispensed milk —and other babies, rocking in corners, wild-eyed and psychotic, after they'd been deprived of contact from birth up to twenty-four months. The psychosis, he demonstrated, was irreversible.

The images are haunting, familiar: the alien, old-man monkey faces with the human eyes, terrorized. Harlow called his monkey isolation chamber the "pit of despair," and the surrogate wire mothers "iron maidens." When the isolated female monkeys were old enough to mate, he had to force them: he called this device the "rape rack." When they delivered their babies, these mothers who had not been mothered often ignored their offspring; sometimes they attacked. Harlow claimed to be studying love.

Harlow's work did hit the intended mark—before his time, psychologists largely believed that love began as a feeding bond and not much else. Harlow proved that a caregiver's emotional connection and physical touch were as vital as food for survival. The stream of Harlow's studies fed into other work being developed by child psychologists like John Bowlby. Harlow bucked contemporary Freudian beliefs about babies' unconscious fantasies and pioneered attachment theory, which posits that babies need to securely attach to a loving, constant caregiver to thrive. These ideas helped transform orphanages from rows of cribs staffed by nurses into family settings and foster care. But the spillage went beyond family psychology and institutional care. Harlow was not only studying love; he was practicing sadism. His abuses were so outrageous that his work effectively spawned the animal rights movement of the twentieth century.

And this is where we get into language. If Harlow hadn't coined the "pit of despair," if "mirror neurons" were called "ventral premotor cortex action recognition signaling" upon their discovery, would the initial streams springing from this work have developed into such rivers?

Harry Harlow was born on Halloween in 1905 as Harry Israel. He changed his name in 1930, after receiving his Ph.D. in psychology from Stanford—a school that, in the 1920s, restricted Jewish enrollment and excluded Jews from fraternities and social offices. His dissertation supervisor promoted eugenics and believed that mental "dullness" came from race and poor breeding.

Harry Israel altered such breeding with a word. Harlow was Harry's father's middle name, a sturdy, Anglo-Saxon bet. It was also a positive echo: the most famous Harlow of that era was another doctor who worked on the brain, a star of then-burgeoning neuroscience. John Martyn Harlow was a nineteenth-century physician who treated Phineas Gage, a railroad foreman who survived the accidental blast of an iron rod, shot directly through his jaw and out through the top of his skull. Gage, remarkably, remained conscious throughout the accident and recovery, and went on to live another twelve years. While Gage continued to walk and talk and think, his disposition was drastically changed: John Harlow wrote that he went from being an affable, well-liked man to being "fitful, irreverent, indulging at times in the grossest profanity."

Gage's left frontal lobe was almost entirely destroyed, and his was the first case to suggest that damage to a specific part of the brain might bring about specific personality changes. Harlow's papers on Gage went on to become fixtures in neurology and psychology curricula, prompting further study. Some connect the later practice of psychosurgery and lobotomies directly to the links Harlow made between brain lesions and character change. The frontal lobe houses the motor cortex where the mirror neurons were found and is also the region for executive control, planning, and behavior control.

That multiple discoveries can bloom from a singular disaster is nothing new. The latter-day Harlow may have mirrored his namesake in this trajectory but he certainly didn't think of his monkey lab as a disaster, or his macaques as anything other than "property I can publish." He never regretted the trauma he imposed. While he studied love, he was known to say of his subjects, "I don't have any love for them . . . How could you like monkeys?"

Still, fortune does have a way of eating its own tail. At the end of his life, Harry Harlow developed Parkinson's, and he died, shaking, like one of his monkeys in a cage.

I FLEW OUT to meet V. S. Ramachandran, strangely enough, ready for a fight. I don't usually approach my interviews with antagonism, but Rama (as he's known) had just published a particularly antagonizing paper. In my field.

For the past twenty years, I've been reporting and writing on transgender communities; my daughter is trans, and I've been partnered with gender variant and trans men. While Ramachandran is known as a behavioral neurologist with a focus on optics, he and a graduate student had just written of a new "neuropsychiatric syndrome" they were calling "alternating gender incongruity." Based on surveys they had conducted online, Ramachandran and his coauthor concluded that their bi-gender respondents had higher rates of bipolar, which they linked to unusual brain hemispheric switching. In reality, the link was unfounded, and what they called a syndrome wasn't new at all but rather a well-documented experience. However, the publication re-pathologized a community and members of my family I've fought long to protect. Suddenly, Rama's attraction to scientific "oddities" touched too close to home. I was supposed to be asking this man about the empathy movement he helped spawn, but I felt more like a mama bear, poised to strike.

At the University of California, San Diego, campus, which is grassy and sprawling, scented with eucalyptus and ocean, I made my way into one of the many concrete buildings dotted about. A graduate student showed me to a chair in the hallway next to an exit sign and some garbage cans; Rama was stuck in traffic. When he finally appeared, he wasn't the boisterous, confident man who appeared on *Charlie Rose* and called mirror neurons "Gandhi neurons," which "dissolved the barrier between me and you." He was thin, much older, and shaking his keys in the lock. I softened.

"Come in," he said, gesturing to me and two students he invited into our talk—one, a medical doctor working on his Ph.D., and another, a visiting scholar on his way to Cambridge, England. The men were young, and doting, and while I first suspected that Rama saw the interview as a bonus lecture for his protégés, I soon realized that he wanted backup.

"It's a famous quote by Darwin—can you please look it up?" Rama said, waving at the scholar. Rama was dressed in a windbreaker and a silky red shirt, open at the neck, with a gold chain dangling a Hindu charm. On his head he wore a paperboy cap, slightly askew, and a full moustache dwarfed his upper lip. He reminded me of the kind of older doo-wop singer you see occasionally on the streets of New York. He talked fast, and he had the tremors, but his style was laid back—an old-school guy who knew things.

I had asked Ramachandran about his role in the mirror neuron boom, the way he'd likened their discovery to DNA, and he scoffed. "That was a throwaway remark, for someone else's website," he said. "It's extraordinary—people don't realize that I've not worked on mirror neurons."

That *was* extraordinary, I pressed, given how much he's had to say about them—in his last book, his TED Talk and in countless interviews, and in his published papers on mirror neurons and human development, apraxia, and autism. Most of Rama's claims, or suppositions, or hypotheses, about mirror neurons have been controversial. And that's what got us to the Darwin quote.

"Try looking under Wikiquote," Rama said to the scholar, who was scrolling through his smartphone. "It's something like, 'False ideas are the lifeblood of science because if they're true they open up a new area of inquiry and if they're false everybody takes delight in destroying them.'"

The scholar didn't find the quote, but I did, later. Darwin didn't call false ideas the lifeblood but rather claimed "false views . . . do little harm." Rama got the other part essentially right, and it's clear he enjoys making trouble. "I usually say very clearly what might be wrong"—and here Rama turned to his students, providing a lesson. "I do a lot of speculation—and you can tell people that. You can tell them: this part of my work is solid, and this part of my work I'm only half sure. But it's a fruitful new approach."

Ramachandran had secured his credibility early in his career with a mirror treatment for phantom limbs and a range of imaginative experiments in behavioral neurology; he's earned honorary doctorates and multiple fellowships and awards. He told his students they needed to establish this kind of sure footing before they could risk such jumps in logic publicly. So, the idea that mirror neurons were responsible for humanity's great leap forward some fifty thousand years ago? "That was totally a jump," he said. He turned back to his students. "If you're going to say something like that, you'd better have your credentials, otherwise people won't listen to you."

The inverse was also true, I thought: if you're famous enough for people to pay attention to you, you'd better be saying something useful—or, at least, not dangerous. The transsexuality suppositions, with their links to bipolar, were downright dangerous—to my mind anyway. I explained my resistance to his scientific methodology: how could he purport to have identified both a new "syndrome" and its potential cause, operating solely from interviews conducted online? I asserted that the trans population overall has been misunderstood and misdiagnosed by the psychiatric community for decades, so relying on self-reports online was in no way an accurate measure of any correlations.

"I guess I should read my students' papers more carefully," Rama said, explaining that his coauthor gathered and produced the results. He liked to give his students free rein to be creative. But then when he saw, during our interview, that the piece had been published in *Medical Hypotheses,* a journal known for far-flung and sometimes offensive theories in the spirit of sparking new research, he recanted: everybody knew, he said, that this was pure speculation. "It's a fishing expedition we're doing—our theories are in the domain of philosophy."

Except when Ramachandran speculates, the media listens. And thus conjecture becomes conclusion. *Discover* picked the story up; so did *Scientific American* and *HuffPo* and the *Daily Mail,* which opened with the line, "Scientists claim to have discovered a new gender of human which is neither male nor female."

The other part of the Darwin quote, which Ramachandran didn't remember or didn't cite, is the opening—before the bit about false views doing little harm. It goes, "False facts are highly injurious to the progress of science, for they often endure long." Darwin didn't live in the internet era, when views could evolve into facts with a few clicks.

This is at the very heart of the mirror neuron debate: as soon as the cells were discovered and theories posited about their role, those suppositions took on the status of fact, and more theories and experiments were built upon that. But many dissenters argue that the mirror neuron edifice—from which books, programs, and centers have sprung—is built on shaky foundations. "There's no direct evidence that mirror neurons are the basis for action understanding; there's no direct evidence for it and lots of evidence against it," says Dr. Gregory Hickok, a professor of cognitive science at the University of California, Irvine, and the author of *The Myth of Mirror Neurons.* "Understanding action" is precisely what Rizzolatti and the Parma team posited the neurons were doing—because they were motor cells that corresponded to movements the monkeys *saw* as well as to movements the monkeys *made.* Hickok notes that in fact these new cells could be doing any number of things (doing basic sensorimotor action planning, for instance). The discovery wasn't the problem, but the inference was, and it launched what Hickok calls "the mirror neuron enterprise."

"In a lot of the psychology papers, the first paragraph assumes mirror neurons are the basis for action understanding. Once you assume that, and if you assume humans have mirror neurons, you can build lots of interesting stories about empathy, language, learning," Hickok said. "But if that foundational assumption is incorrect then the whole house of cards falls."

At the beginning, mirror neuron skeptics complained that the cells had never been found in humans: monkey proof didn't equal human proof. The mirror neurons in macaques are a very specific subset of individual cells discovered only by sticking micro-thin electrodes into many neurons and then picking them out one by one. Scientists couldn't do this in humans because they couldn't go around sawing open skulls. Until, in 2009, they could.

NEUROSCIENCE LABORATORIES, despite their sexy sci-fi implications, tend to look like any other college department: people sit at desks and work on computers. fMRI scanners, EEG machines—all the tools that actually peer beneath the skull—are locked away in other rooms or other buildings for their short interludes with subjects. Most of the work happens after scans or recordings are gathered. Scientists correct for noise and motion, compare variance, and analyze data points before they come up with anything that looks like the Sno-Cone–colored photographs they publish.

I had been to the UCLA Brain Mapping Center years back, when my first wife, a neurophysicist, was getting her Ph.D. there. That was before it became the site where mirror neurons were first identified in humans. The place was exactly as I remembered it: skylights, polished cement floors, butter-yellow couches, and closed doors, behind which lab directors sat at blonde, wraparound desks with their laptops. I met with Dr. Marco Iacoboni, who directs the lab, and the graduate students who found the human mirror neurons. He sat at one of these desks, spotless save for his computer and a framed photo of Roger Federer he had won at an auction.

Iacoboni speaks quickly and with an accent; he's from Rome. He was surprised when people demanded evidence of mirror neurons in humans: they don't require such replication in other animal discoveries. After all, he said, the whole ethical justification for animal research is undermined if you can't make human inferences. Still, when epilepsy patients at UCLA had single-cell electrodes implanted for pre-surgery recordings, Iacoboni's graduate student Roy Mukamel went to their beds and had them perform similar tasks to the original macaques in Italy.

They found mirror neurons, but the parallels weren't perfect. In fact, Mukamel and his team saw mirror neurons also in non-motor regions. "They were in the entorhinal cortex, which is a part of the brain that is important for memory, visual processing," Iacoboni said, adding that when he first saw the data, he couldn't believe it. But then he realized mirroring went much further than merely repeating an action. "When I see you grabbing a cup of coffee, I not only activate my motor plans to derive the same motor use to grab a cup of coffee. I also have all these memory neurons in the medial temporal lobe," he said. "These memory neurons remember the neural trace of myself grabbing a cup of coffee. Which in turn invokes all these memories associated with the smell of the coffee, my dopamine release when I'm anticipating drinking the coffee. All these things are part of a very rich form of empathizing with others, it's very foundational."

But what about the idea that Hickok raises? All we can really tell about mirror neurons is that they discharge. How did Iacoboni *know* their role in the process he described?

"Of course, it's very difficult to completely prove it; that's a very high bar to set," Iacoboni said. He opened and closed his laptop and smiled. He was a believer. He had written *Mirroring People: The Science of Empathy and How We Connect with Others* a few years back —the first book in English to explain mirror neurons and their potential to a lay audience. Iacoboni said that the basic reason that he, Rizzolatti, and now many others believed that mirror neurons formed the basis for action understanding was that that is simply how it felt, inside, experientially. "We think that's what they're doing because of a phenomenological experience."

In other words, all this science is based on a hunch — the intuitive sense that when "I" watch "you," I don't cognitively, logically, think through your actions. Rather, I restage my own memory of this action (and experience its attendant emotional associations) in an internal neural map of myself. Iacoboni nodded: yes, this depiction of mirror neuron function was intuitive. But it was only a start.

"Our analogy is that you have a house. The house is empathy. Mirroring is not the whole house, but it's the foundation," he said. "On top of the house, you can build other things, much more complex things."

The mirroring process, he thinks, is very simple: babies do it right out of the womb when they copy tongue movements and other facial expressions. More complex imitation is built on this mirroring, and learning can be built on that. Iacoboni says humans imitate one another unconsciously, automatically, though some do it more than others. There are now studies that show the more often a person imitates, the more empathic she'll be in social situations. This, he suggests, could indicate mirror neurons are a starting line. "It tells us that in fact the way we get into the minds of others is by simulating or imitating or reenacting what they do."

THE DAY I WENT to visit Ramachandran in San Diego, his office looked like that of an eccentric Victorian scientist. There were jars of brains scattered about and a plaster cast of a saber-toothed tiger skeleton perched atop his desk. Like his surroundings, Rama was more colorful than Dr. Iacoboni in his response to the mirror neuron debate: "All the objections they've raised are nonsense: they're confounding mechanism, which is what we're trying to understand with mirror neurons, with description, which is the theory of other minds. It's like saying if you know about the feces that come out from the food you're eating you don't need to know about the liver, the pancreas. It's a straw man."

But the straw man's gaining weight and heft. The people looking to disprove mirror neurons are, still, studying mirror neurons. And the believers, like Iacoboni, are exploring what they call "mirror systems"—psychological experiments on empathy replete with whole-brain scans that, as of now, can't isolate images of single neurons, mirror or otherwise. Ramachandran and his lab have taken scanning and the brain out of the equation entirely; they're just looking at empathic exchanges.

"The discovery of the mirror neurons led us to ask this question in the first place," Ramachandran said, explaining a current experiment wherein subjects with obsessive-compulsive traits are asked to witness an experimenter touch disgusting (and unbeknownst to them, false) things like feces and vomit. The OCD subjects then instruct the experimenter to wash his hands in a specific way or perform a ritual—and the subjects reportedly feel relief. This, Ramachandran suggests, could have treatment implications: OCD patients, rather than performing their own elaborate rituals in their own lives, could perhaps watch shorter and shorter videos of ritual performances until the need disappears.

And maybe that's the point of all this: mirror neuron science may be misguided, but it's given us a new place to look. Iacoboni is excited about the cross-pollination that empathy research has yielded —between neuroscience and psychology, neuroscience and philosophy. He's been talking with anthropologists and authors to understand the ways they think about empathy and then talking with engineers about designing brain implants to scan interactions in real time.

"Right now we study brains in isolation. Ideally, you want to study brains that are interacting," Iacoboni said. This means developing a now-distant technology, as well as transforming the way scientists, and a lot of us, think. He looked around his corner office: it has frosted windows, so he couldn't look out, and no one could look in. "Academics seem to spend a lot of time in their offices, thinking and writing in isolation, so that's the dominant model in academia. In fact, our brain is shaped by our social interactions. If I strip all my social relationships out of myself, nothing is left."

And if I break down all the articles and books and news reports and look at the programs and departments and experts they've spawned, this is the essential message of the mirror neurons: we are social creatures. It's not that this idea is new or revolutionary; it's that it bucks up against the Darwinian-individualist ethos that's dominated for generations. Mirror neurons invited an about-face. They invited us to think not about how we get ahead but how we get along.

While I welcome this shift, this newfound recognition that we human beings are destined for relation rather than almighty independence, something sticks in my throat when I hear about new empathy studies. Something closes in. Sometimes it's the marketing, or the commodification of kindness, the empathy-with-a-goal that bothers me. But it's also something fundamental in the language and approach, something that, despite the squabbling over empathy semantics and definitions in academia, hasn't been defined or theorized enough in society at large. Empathy hasn't grown up. Mirrors, after all, are the root metaphor here, and mirrors don't let us see other people. They only bounce us right back to ourselves.

2

Teach Your Children Well

Once we've moved beyond the basics of how empathy works, via simulation theory or mirror neurons, we begin to think about what empathy *is*. If it is indeed a skill, then it's something that can be acquired, mastered, and quantified. It's something you can put on and take off again, like any skill you learn. But if it's something more inborn, like an identity or an orientation, then empathy's a way of being in the world, a way of inherently understanding the other.

In broad brushstrokes, these are the two ways empathy is configured — as a skill or an orientation. It's something that we *do* or something that we *are*. And, as with many things that we're trying to culturally disentangle, we make children our lab rats.

But first we sound the alarm bells. For the past thirty years, researchers have been asking college students, the people who have just stepped out of childhood, to rate themselves on something called the Interpersonal Reactivity Index. The students self-report their own levels of empathy. They answer positively or negatively to statements like, "I often have tender, concerned feelings for people less fortunate than me," and "I try to look at everybody's side of a disagreement before I make a decision." The last study, conducted on fourteen thousand students, showed 75 percent rated themselves less empathic than students thirty years ago — spawning a flurry of concerned articles about the sorry state of kids today.

Rick Weissbourd is one of these concerned people. Weissbourd is on the faculty at Harvard's Kennedy School of Education and Kennedy School of Government, and for the last decade, he's been taking surveys of schoolchildren all over the country — asking them what matters in their lives now and in the future.

"It appears that achievement just keeps getting more and more important in many middle- and upper-class communities; it has almost an epidemic quality to it," Weissbourd said to me over the phone. In 2014, his group at Harvard surveyed more than fifteen thousand middle- and high-school kids from diverse backgrounds. They asked the kids to rank happiness (defined as feeling good most of the time), high achievement, and caring for others.

Eighty percent chose happiness or achievement first — the same percentage that said their parents also valued one of those aspects of personal success over caring about other people. While neither the college study nor Weissbourd's study defines empathy per se, and both swap in a lot of other words like "caring" or "concern," they signal a level of renewed attention to the ways our kids tune in to the others around them. And while experts may squabble over whether empathy itself is inborn or learned, its decline, they feel, is undoubtedly cultural.

"I felt this in my own community and with my own kids and in the parenting culture I was in — there was a lot of attention to how kids felt about themselves moment to moment, a hyper-attentiveness to getting needs met, and organizing around kids, and not enough attention to other people," Weissbourd said. "At other moments in history there was much more attention to preparing children for citizenship and participation in the common good."

His remarks harmonize with the widespread lament that we are more isolated than ever by our screens, and that the interactions we have through them are superficial and false. Many, of course, argue the opposite: that the internet is evidence of our ever-increasing global connection. Both positions are so broad, they tip right over, and almost anyone could argue either side. What's incontestable is this: we're spending more of our daylight hours linking up with more people than ever before, and more people are interested in watching us do it. Experientially, this might feel like empathy. Empathy, by some definitions, is being seen.

The first time I shopped for dog food online and then saw an ad for pet supplies in my newsfeed moments later, I was startled. Now this is entirely commonplace. In a few years, the cookies we scatter for advertisers to follow will seem as innocuous as their name. Companies called things like Emotient and Affectiva have developed facial recognition software to detect our fleeting micro-expressions as we scroll through our days. A smirk of recognition at a couple arguing in a YouTube video will prompt an ad for local marriage counseling; a frown at bare midriffs will cue up conservative clothes.

It may sound Big Brother to turn the video camera on oneself, but marketers are betting we'll do it: as of early 2015, there were more than a hundred patents in the works for facial emotion recognition software. After all, billions of us already willingly supply, or numbly ignore, the personal data we give away for free: our location, our friends, our likes, our private messages.

As we wear straps on our wrists that count our steps, and glasses on our faces that track where we look, and as these devices remit data back to the corporations that made them so they can sell us even better straps and glasses to guide us to sites with ever-more-personalized products, we may even like it. Surveillance, as it's normalized, can feel like devotion.

Whistle-blowers and reporters worry about the National Security Agency prying into our emails and phone calls, but I teach at a major university and every year, my students are less and less concerned. It's happening anyway, they figure, and they're accustomed to being looked at. Privacy is not their burden; what they fear is anonymity.

The umbrella term for all the electronic sensors that pick up our expressions and moods and patterns and preferences and feed them back to corporations to sell us stuff is "empathic computing." The fifth international workshop for empathic computing was held in Sydney, Australia. Program committee members hailed from Japan, the Philippines, France, Vietnam, Italy, Thailand, Belgium, and the United States. Organizers wanted papers on intention recognition, wearable or implantable sensor integration, and data fusion in ambient spaces, among other topics. One interesting implantable device is a pill with a sensor inside, developed by Motorola (owned by Google) and already approved by the U.S. Food and Drug Administration. When the pill mixes with the stomach's gastric juices, the sensor flips on to authenticate a person's electronic devices, rendering passwords (and, presumably, a person's freedom of unmonitored movement) obsolete. A key executive and spokesperson for the pill comes directly from the Department of Defense.

At MIT, the empathic computing group is working on building a cloud system for collecting longitudinal biophysiological feedback and on reinventing retail experiences using individual skin conductors, among dozens of other projects. Their empathic car design uses existing technologies to sense a driver's emotional state (via heart-rate, grasping, palm sweat, etc.) and alter music, temperature, GPS voice, and colors in the dashboard to match it.

As we increasingly expect our houses, our cars, our phones, and the pills we swallow to cater directly to our moment-by-moment wishes, we may feel more mirrored, more empathically met, even if only by products and websites. We may also, consciously or less so, feel that a finely tuned sensitivity is an important skill to cultivate in this shifting market that values individualized targeting and social networking over all else. And this might be the disconnect that Rick Weissbourd noticed when he surveyed students all across the country. We're *saying* we want our kids to learn empathy, but we are still *acting* like achievement matters more. If the empathy we're swimming in is market-driven or achievement-based, this makes a sudden kind of sense. We'll try to fix the empathy gap with an achievable, teachable skill you can learn. In the classroom.

Ashoka is a multimillion-dollar nonprofit with a branch called the "Empathy Initiative." Their stated goal is for every schoolchild across the globe to learn empathy. This sounds grandiose, but a big part of their strategy is to draw upon and connect the best practices of the many hundreds of schools and organizations that are already building empathy curricula—primarily in North America, but on other continents too. I talked with the founding director of the Empathy Initiative, Danielle Goldstone, before I had thought through any of these ideas about digital culture. I just called to ask about the focus of her nonprofit, and she headed right for the internet.

"The world where we educate people through repetition, to be factory workers, that world is going very quickly as hierarchies come down as we all work in more networked ways," Goldstone said, emphasizing that Ashoka's long history of funding social entrepreneurs working all over the world gives them a unique perspective on our international, interconnected historical moment. "There are so many different cultures colliding now, you're constantly having to work with diverse groups of people to get anything done. Empathy is the essential skill to solve problems."

And what are the problems? "Right now," she said, "the unemployment rate globally is going up—and we have companies that have positions they can't fill with the people coming out of schools. Companies are saying we need people that can collaborate, people that are creative—people who can innovate. In the customer service world this is a huge conversation; empathy is an important part of customer service."

When Goldstone said this, I immediately pictured a customer-service operator with a headset telephone fielding calls; sure, I thought, it would be great if telemarketers were in better moods. Later, of course, I realized, "customer service" now captures the universe of our wired lives: from surveillance, to tracking, to targeting, to capturing customers, and back out to other marketers in endless growing loops.

I asked Goldstone whether teaching empathy to kids, then, was about helping them to make money. No, she said, but the goal is to make everybody powerful. And there isn't anything wrong with wanting success *and* empathy.

"This is where Rick and I have a lot of discussions," she said, meaning Rick Weissbourd, at Harvard. Ashoka recently hired Weissbourd and his nonprofit, Making Caring Common, to compile an analysis of school-based empathy programs in the United States. "I think for Rick, it's about moral development—teaching empathy for empathy's sake. I always tell him I'm really excited that we live in a world that values success *and* values empathy. Companies are clamoring for this skill."

This is where we hit the split in the understanding of empathy itself. *Is* empathy a skill to be optimized or is it a moral inclination to be nurtured?

When I spoke with Weissbourd, he talked directly about this division in child education—and it's a big one. It turns out almost everyone's on board the empathy train, but there are deep divisions about where the train is headed.

On one side are the Social and Emotional Learning (SEL) groups. If you have a child currently enrolled in a U.S. school, it's likely she's had some SEL curricula sprinkled in among the reading and math. Nobody knows exactly how many programs are running, but the U.S. Department of Education recently recommended SEL, and many schools use it to comply with the anti-bullying laws now enacted in forty-nine states.

Empathy is a key component of Social and Emotional Learning—alongside managing emotions, setting goals, and maintaining relationships. SEL is designed for every year from pre-K through high school—and its advocates point to the more than two hundred studies that show that SEL kids have fewer conduct problems and better grades. These outcomes highlight the SEL approach: it's competence-based and goal-oriented. Kids are expected to learn something, do something, and get something for themselves out of it all. Empathy, in this rubric, is a *skill*. As Goldstone said, "Empathy is a capacity we all innately have, but one of our principles is to treat it like playing the piano. If you practice it and practice, you're going to get good at it."

The people on the other side of the education train — the Rick Weissbourds of the world — view empathy through a completely different lens. They see empathy primarily as a *moral quality,* a critical value that distinctly shapes how one moves through the world. "It isn't just about developing the skill of empathy — it's about developing an identity that is organized around other people," Weissbourd said. "People like Nelson Mandela or Martin Luther King — they don't talk about their acts as a choice but something they had to do as a reflex — as part of their identity."

For Weissbourd, you begin with deep moral instruction and with moral relationships — the tools and skills are secondary. You model for children and teach them that other people matter; you provide them with that core and intrinsic value. From there, they're motivated to learn more empathy — because it fits with an identity they already have. Proponents of this approach often refer to it as "moral development" or "character education."

Empathy, when articulated as a skill, can be both cognitive and emotional, but it's essentially about perspective-taking, which can be measured and discussed, dissected and mapped. Empathy-as-identity is trickier: by its very definition it's personal and thus both bound by an individual's psychology and rendered limitless by the infinite capacity of human connection. And so, the educators' question is essentially everybody's question in this violent and fragmented world: do we want to be better, do better, or do we simply want to understand?

· · ·

MARY GORDON IS ANOTHER major player in empathy education. Her program, Roots of Empathy (ROE), is now running in every province in Canada, has launched in several European countries and New Zealand, and is just starting to tiptoe into a few schools in the United States. Gordon herself is an old-timer in the field. She created ROE the same year that Rizzolatti was discovering his mirror neurons and the empathy vortex was gathering momentum. (UC Berkeley's Greater Good Science Center called ROE the "world's most effective empathy teaching program.") She's a small woman in her sixties, with blonde hair and green eyes that widen when she tells a sad or moving story, which is often. I met with Gordon at New York University, where she was giving a talk to the Stern School of Business. Business schools, she said, have lately grown very interested in her work. Which is funny because her primary teaching tool is a baby under one year old.

"I call it 'the tiny teacher,'" Gordon said, explaining that despite her curriculum planning book's six-hundred-page length, the essential lesson of ROE is simple: bring a baby into a classroom and let the children observe, ask questions, and reflect on their own feelings or similar experiences. "We're trying to help them find the humanity in that baby, and it takes about five minutes."

Roots of Empathy isn't strictly SEL or moral education — though it has elements of both — but rather twenty-seven set lesson plans, targeted to different ages, from pre-K through middle school. Here's how it works: every three weeks, the same baby and her parent will show up at a classroom, and the kids will gather around, singing her songs, noticing her milestones, and observing the parent's attachment. In the weeks before and after visits, they'll talk about what happened, how they felt, or make the baby small gifts — like construction paper trees, with wishes for her future scrawled on the leaves.

"We're very much working on the notion that little children are huge, keen observers of humanity. In that moment when they find the humanity in the baby, we flip everything that happens back to the child. When was a time that you felt like that? It's helping the children learn what I call emotional literacy," Gordon said, speaking softly and quickly and holding my gaze. People think she has an Irish accent, and she sprinkles her speech with words like "wee" and "grand," but she was raised in Newfoundland and went to school with Irish nuns. "It's like a laboratory, almost, but it's a laboratory of melded hearts, not just inspection. It's reflection. It's engagement. It's interdependence versus the ridiculous, dangerous independence that we so lionize in North American culture."

THE BISHOP JOHN T. WALKER SCHOOL FOR BOYS recently brought in Roots of Empathy, and when Anthony Davis, a site coordinator at the school, first heard about the program, he was skeptical. The school is located in Washington, D.C.'s infamous Ward 8, the poorest in the district, where 70 percent of elementary-aged kids are not proficient in reading and half of the dropouts do so before high school. Out of every one hundred kids who do enter high school, only thirteen will graduate. Davis thought that the kind of "ridiculous, dangerous independence" that Mary Gordon snubbed might be necessary in a neighborhood like this.

"I was worried it [ROE] would make the boys soft, given the environments they come from," Davis said to me when he met me at my taxi in front of the school, which was housed in the corner of an apartment complex. He talked with the driver about picking me up after my visit; he didn't think it was safe for me to just stand around in the parking lot and wait. In one hand he held a tote bag filled with a baby booster pillow, some plush toys, and the ubiquitous green blanket used in every ROE encounter. Despite his misgivings, Davis had become a ROE instructor. "The principal wanted somebody to volunteer, and I didn't think anybody else would be so into it," he confessed with a little half-shrug.

The Bishop Walker School is very small: only eighty-four students total for kindergarten through fifth grade spread over two separate sites. "This used to be a junior high for girls," Davis said, as he showed me around a multipurpose room where the kids can get free breakfast, lunch, and dinner; a small chapel; and a bright, cozy library with orange walls and a green shag rug and cushions scattered about. On display were several books about Barack Obama and the civil rights movement. Three classrooms and some offices fill out the remainder of the school for the thirty-one boys in the upper three grades who go here. The school is private but tuition-free, as it's specifically targeted to low-income families east of the Anacostia River.

In the stairwell, Davis was accosted by a throng of boys headed outside for recess. They all wore khakis and blue oxford button-downs. Some had on sweatshirts emblazoned with the school logo.

"Mr. Davis! Mr. Davis!" they shouted. One boy jumped in for a head butt-cum-hug, and there were hand slaps and squeezes all around.

"My dad says I've been losing weight!" one kid said, a triumphant grin on his face.

"My man!" Davis replied, and high-fived him.

Suddenly, inexplicably, they were all shouting about their weight-loss programs.

"I've been running!" one kid said.

"And I haven't been eating so much!"

Over the boys' heads, Davis shot me a quizzical look. These were fifth graders, boys gazing headlong into the middle distance of adolescence. They knew their bodies, and the way the world would relate to them, were about to change dramatically, and maybe they were managing that impending shift in whatever way they could. Or maybe they were just being eleven.

Anyway, for now, for a little bit longer, they were children safely ensconced in a school that clearly cherished them. Its hallways were decorated with their artwork and with quilts that displayed their handprints as they grew from year to year. In the open space be-tween classrooms, where Davis spread the green blanket for ROE, I saw a writing prompt pinned to the wall. It read, "Great writers write about what is important to them and these are small moments. Try writing a seed story, not a watermelon story."

We were waiting for the third-grade class, which was led—like all of the classes at Bishop John T. Walker—by a teacher with both a B.A. and a master's from top universities. The faculty bio page is littered with Yales, Howards, Morehouses, and Stanfords. The Roots of Empathy mom, Lakishia Freeman, sat patiently on a plastic child's chair, her baby Faith bouncing and grinning on her knee. Her other daughter, two-year-old Nyla, was running around looking for her older brother, who she just knew was behind one of the closed doors; she had seen him peep out a moment before. ROE doesn't pay its instructors or its parents or offer any form of child-care, so siblings like Nyla just get folded into the lesson however they fit.

"I used to work as a bus driver, but I gave it up when the daycare was costing more than my mortgage," Freeman said to me. She's thirty-five and soft all over: soft features, soft voice, soft gestures with her kids. Her middle son, Justin, was a fifth grader at Bishop Walker, and when he came home talking about the ROE baby who visited, she figured she could volunteer, once she had Baby Faith. "I like answering the boys' questions, I like the developmental stage they're at."

The developmental stage, it turned out, was a crossroads be-tween earnest and goofball. The class of ten third graders left their classroom in a solemn straight line and spaced themselves evenly around the green blanket. Freeman stood, holding Faith outward, and circled the room, letting each boy squeeze Faith's foot as they sang a dirge-lullaby called "Hello, Baby Faith, How Are You." When the song was over, they dropped to the floor, all elbows and knees and giggles. The ones farthest from the baby played some sort of secret handshake/pattycake game with each other, the closer ones squeezed in toward the baby.

Nyla, the two-year-old, looked panicked. She wedged herself in between the boys and her sister and began pushing them roughly away.

"Na-Na, it's okay," Lakishia soothed, as Mr. Davis asked the class what they noticed about Baby Faith as they sang her the song.

"She was smiling," one said.

"Yeah, but she was smiling weird, like happy-sad."

"Look, she's eating the pillow!" one kid shrieked, pointing at Faith, who was propped up on the booster Davis had brought.

Lakishia explained that Faith was teething. Today's ROE theme was "emotions," and Davis tried to steer everybody back on track. He asked Freeman about the things that made Baby Faith sad.

"If she's hungry, or if she hears a noise she's unfamiliar with," she answered. Baby Faith did not look sad. She was staring intently at a boy who was wagging a cloth book in front of her face. Some boys pointed this out.

"She looks focused."

"She's focused on Daryl!"

One boy, positioned so he couldn't see Faith's face, asked, "Why is she bald at the back of her head?"

Baldness notwithstanding, Faith was exhibiting the developmentally appropriate empathy for her age group. So were the boys. And so was Nyla, who was now leaning against Davis, warily watching the exchange with her sister, judging whether to step back in and give another shove.

Martin L. Hoffman is a well-known developmental psychologist who laid out the four basic stages of empathy development. The first he calls "global empathy," which appears in a child's first year of life, and it's essentially involuntary mirroring or matching whatever emotion she sees. Global empathy is the reason a baby will cry when she hears another baby crying — and why Faith was imitating

Daryl's happy, focused expression as he wagged a toy in front of her face.

The second stage is called "egocentric empathy," and it emerges in the second year: Nyla's age. By two years old, kids like Nyla will offer empathic help to others, but it's of the egocentric variety; they provide only what they themselves imagine would be comforting. This is why Nyla pushed the boys away when her sister seemed perfectly content with their ministrations. *Nyla* wouldn't have wanted those kids in her business, so she expected Baby Faith wouldn't either.

In another year, Nyla will realize that people can have feelings that differ from her own, a stage simply called "empathy for another's feelings." The kids in third grade were well into this stage, as they knew Baby Faith, and Nyla, and all the kids that sat around the blanket were separate people with separate interior landscapes. Articulating the features of these landscapes, however, takes both a kind of attention and vocabulary, and it's these skills Davis is trying to boost.

"If Baby Faith cries, does that mean she's bad?" he asked.

"Noooo!" most of the kids shouted in unison. They knew the answer to this. "She's communicating."

Baby Faith was not crying; she was laughing at Daryl. When I talked with Mary Gordon, she said ROE instructors always hope that babies will cry during a visit, so the kids can describe their own experiences of sadness, as well as other feelings that may crop up. She calls this "building an emotional alphabet." The other important element to crying is the soothing; ROE kids can witness parents bonding with their babies and meeting their needs. "If the children sitting around the green blanket weren't lucky enough to have a secure attachment relationship when they were little," Gordon said, "well, now they have a picture of one."

My stomach dropped a little when Mary said that; it struck me as particularly cruel. ROE suddenly seemed like a more intense version of watching happy families on TV and wondering what was wrong in your own house, except this time the haunting scene was being enacted with people you knew, when you were surrounded by all your friends. I asked her if exhibiting this "attachment relationship" ever created a sense of longing or loss in the kids.

Mary looked at me levelly. "It doesn't create it, it's there." And then she claimed that it was better to address these painful feelings, at least in a classroom setting. "Would you rather not be in touch with who you are in your pain and be oblivious and resentful?"

This, I imagined, required a pretty high level of attenuation from the instructor (who had a room full of kids and a baby to watch) and sophistication on the part of the kid. In the Washington classroom I observed, some of the kids watched Freeman closely as she tenderly stroked Faith's head or scooted her up on the pillow. Others seemed to intentionally look away — or maybe they were just more interested in playing the hand games with their classmates. When Davis engaged them in questions about sadness, some took the bait, but others shifted the conversation.

"When I'm playing a game on my grandmother's phone, I have to let my brother play," one boy with a round face complained, curiously. Because there are no wrong answers in Roots of Empathy, the teacher let him continue about the injustice for several minutes. "I try to teach him how, but he won't listen to me."

Hoffman's fourth stage of development can track in a bit later than third grade. While the D.C. kids can recognize that Baby Faith is a separate person with separate needs and feelings, they can't yet consistently grasp the ways different people have different life circumstances than their own. So there's the rub. Faith's happiness and close bond with her mother could kick up seemingly inconsistent or confusing feelings of frustration and envy ("I hate sharing the game with my brother") just when a kid doesn't have the tools to understand that everybody's parents and family circumstances are different. This stage of empathic development gets deepened at an even later age, sometime around twelve, when kids can feel a kind of empathy for distressed groups (like homeless people or war veterans).

Experiencing poor early attachment isn't just about feeling confused or sad when you witness good attachment like Faith's. Poor attachment means you can have trouble empathizing at all. I asked Gordon about this, about the kids in her classrooms who may have been neglected or abused in their own infancy, and she agreed—studies show that babies who don't have a secure, consistent relationship with their caregivers are less able to tune in to the emotional lives of others. And this, she says, robs you of sustainable relationships throughout life. Which, in turn, robs you of an understanding of yourself.

"Loneliness, I think, is one of our biggest poverties. There's a violence to loneliness, you know," she said. Her biggest concern, however, isn't that children in her programs could turn out to be aggressors or bullies, which is the emphasis of a lot of the social and emotional learning programs. Her focus is empathy—and for those who can't feel it, they can at least begin to identify feelings within themselves. Hence, they work on the emotional alphabet. "To develop empathy, you can have self-empathy first. It's important that you understand yourself."

MARY GORDON'S ALSO working off the basic folk definition of empathy, meaning she's helping kids stand in another's shoes—to emotionally feel some experience and cognitively talk about it. Babies, who don't even wear shoes yet, make easy test subjects because their emotions seem fairly primary: angry, sad, happy, curious. This obviously gets more complicated as we empathize with older people, who exhibit more layered responses to more layered life circumstances.

And here's where we begin to find more divergent definitions of empathy. Dominic McIver Lopes, a professor of philosophy at the University of British Columbia, who comes mainly from an art and aesthetics tradition and is the past president of the American Society for Aesthetics, claims that nobody *feels* empathy because empathy is not a feeling. He says it doesn't belong on a list with anger, pity, joy, and so on, though experiencing empathy always involves one or more of the emotions we're picking up from the other person. Lopes likens empathy to a skill, and the breadth of one's empathic skill will be limited by the emotions one has experienced oneself. For instance, if you've never experienced shattering loneliness, murderous rage, or even ecstatic delight, you won't be able to empathize with these states in another.

This, of course, makes me think of cross-cultural empathy and how much a person can truly hope to empathize with someone in radically different circumstances who, because of cultural conditioning, has felt the contours of her life in radically different ways. If empathy is not a feeling but rather an ability to adopt another's perspective (emotionally, cognitively, affectively, and so on), then this perspective too is circumscribed by both where we stand and how similar another's shoes are to our own.

RESEARCH SHOWS THAT we do, generally, have more empathy for people who we believe share similar values or come from similar backgrounds than we do for people who are unfamiliar. This has troubling implications for advocates (like me) of more empathy in other kinds of public spheres like, for instance, the courtroom. One study of mock trials showed that a jury's sentencing recommendations were influenced by how "sad" the victim or defendant seemed. The jury doled out harsher sentences when the victim was sad and lighter ones when the defendant was sad. Another study shows people had more empathic responses to pictures of faces in their same ethnic group (measured by physiological response and viewing time). It's not that we can't conjure empathy for a wide range of beings—and even nonbeings; people feel empathy for computers and cars and plastic dinosaurs too. We just fool ourselves if we think all empathy is created equal.

These kinds of studies, however, are often examining rather simplistic, instinctive, or lower-level forms of empathy. It's the kind of empathy that happens almost automatically: you smile, I smile; you fall, I wince. Higher-level empathy, the kind the kids were practicing at the Bishop John T. Walker School, involves the imagination. Higher-level empathy is, at root, taking on a new perspective.

Modern accounts of perspective-taking put it into three camps:

A. Self-focused (how would this feel for *me* to experience your situation?)

B. Other-focused (how would this feel for *you* to experience your situation?)

C. A combination of A and B, either sequentially or simultaneously

At first blush, B might intuitively seem the most empathic or generous, but several people who write about empathy argue against this approach. Peter Goldie was a chair in philosophy at the University of Manchester and the coeditor of one of the best collections of philosophical and psychological essays on empathy (he died in 2011). He claimed that imagining your way into another's mind in order to experience his feelings *as that person* essentially swallows up his agency. Better, he wrote, to keep the separation between self and other distinct. Go ahead and imagine the feelings and their context, but as you would feel them. It's probably more honest: you only have your own brain to draw from anyhow. Recognizing your limitations keeps you listening.

As a writer who reports on subjects with lives and stories vastly different from my own, though, I feel a responsibility to embrace version B. I *am* other-focused in my empathy. When I write about street kids, for instance—and I've written about them a lot—I do try to inhabit them, in my way. I've never lived on the street, but I don't try to imagine how I would feel with one pair of jeans and a terrible secret. Instead, I listen very carefully to that individual child, absorbing as much as I can of both her verbal and nonverbal storytelling, slipping into her world until she softens that secret and I think I can feel, for an instant, what it's like to have her pulse beating in my skin. But maybe this is hubris. Or maybe it's stealing or lying or both.

I hate the idea of robbing anyone of their agency, and good reporters are trained to guard against this always. But I'm not sure the A-B-C model is entirely accurate—though, to be fair, it is a model, and reductive by nature. It gives us a jumping-off point. For me, higher-level empathy is about a cognitive grasp of context—a person's self-stated background and longings and traumas that shaped them—but after this, or just before, there is contagion. This emotional transfer, the zap of feeling you intuit but don't necessarily transfer to an intellectual processing place, is considered lower-level, but it doesn't go away just because you can imagine yourself in another's context. (To be clear, Goldie and anti-"other-focused" empathy philosophers aren't opposed to gathering context, just to presuming knowledge of another's lived experience within it.) These higher and lower levels work in tandem; you feel your way into thinking and think your way into feeling. Self and other do become blurred—for moments, but not forever. This fleeting merger gives empathy its resonance; the separation, its articulation. In this way, empathy is not unlike love.

NEL NODDINGS WRITES about ideal empathy as a kind of receptivity; she describes the standard notion of empathy wherein one projects oneself into another "peculiarly rational, western, masculine." Noddings is a social psychologist whose work, in the tradition of Carol Gilligan, is primarily in care ethics, which came about in the 1980s and emphasized a more relational style in the ethical treatment of others, utilizing both reason and emotion, as opposed to abstract rules and "fairness." I'm not so sure about gendering particular empathic approaches, but I do like the idea of receptivity over projection. The focus shifts into tuning the instrument: listening better, hearing more.

Noddings's version also gestures toward empathy with a moral core — a vision Rick Weissbourd from Making Caring Common also shares. For Weissbourd, we learn to be empathic to strengthen the fibers of our community fabric, to care about others because that's the right thing to do. For Mary Gordon at Roots of Empathy, we learn empathy to build our own individual emotional vocabularies, to connect with others to reduce personal and interpersonal violence. For Danielle Goldstone at Ashoka, empathy builds skills toward success. For me, I like empathy because it's interesting — it's the only way to be intimate and expansive at once.

So what are we talking about when we talk about empathy? I worry about the messianic, colonialist undertones of U.S. organizations that promise to teach every child, the world over, about empathy, when people are of course already practicing empathy in their own culturally determined ways. One telling survey asked parents and teachers of preschoolers to list the top thing children should learn in preschool. In Japan, for instance, the number one answer was already "sympathy/empathy/ concern for others." (In the United States, the top choice was "self-reliance/self-confidence.") The basic definition of empathy in Japanese, *omoiyari,* is somewhat different, however, because it extends past feeling and into action. It means "the ability and willingness to feel what others are feeling, to vicariously experience the pleasure or pain that they are undergoing, and to help them satisfy their wishes."

Mary Gordon herself says that empathy can't be taught — but it can be learned. Essentially, we are empathic toward others if others (our families, our teachers, our communities) are modeling it. The motivation for empathy, and the type of empathy we practice, is the type we see. Which naturally can change when our environment changes.

Gordon and Roots of Empathy advocates hope that a nine-month journey with a baby and a green blanket will be enough of an environmental change to bolster a child's empathy. So far, there have been no longitudinal studies, though Gordon and her team are working on it. What they have demonstrated is that kids in schools with Roots of Empathy show reduced aggression and increased pro-social behavior immediately following the program, and that these outcomes are maintained for three years. When I look around a school like Bishop Walker, with its bright paintings by students on the walls, its giant floor rug depicting all the American states, and a teacher like Anthony Davis, who plays ball outdoors with the kids in one of the most impoverished neighborhoods in the nation, it's hard to tell which positive input is affecting which positive outcome. But I do know a baby named Faith can't hurt.

3

The Experimental Self

Several decades before schoolchildren were learning about empathy from babies, adults were taking trainings in empathic listening. Nonviolent Communication, or NVC, may be the most recognizable empathy brand. People in more than sixty-five countries have studied the three steps: self-empathy, receiving empathically, and expressing honestly. The basic methodology to NVC hasn't changed much since psychologist Marshall Rosenberg launched it in the late 1960s, except in the last decade, they've added more emphasis to the self-empathy component. If we really are, as a culture, becoming more self-centered, this isn't surprising at all.

The general NVC class lasts for eight weeks, but because I live in New York City, where everything happens faster, I could only find a three-hour crash course called "Empathic Communication." After I signed up and schlepped my way through a cold November snow to an address several blocks from a subway line, my first task was to muster empathy for an instructor who was thirty-five minutes late. In a classroom painted in shades of pistachio and lemon, three other students and I chatted about why we were there and chomped on walnuts someone had placed in a bowl. We were above an Ayurvedic restaurant, and the room smelled like lentil stew.

"I'm here to learn boundaries," said a woman named Molly with long, dark hair and bright makeup. Molly was a flight attendant, and she complained bitterly about her passengers; they were forever treating her like a waitress, or worse, a servant. I expected her to say she wanted to understand travelers' motivations better, or some other empathy-related line of thought, but no: Molly was taking an empathy class to learn to shut people out. I liked her immediately.

Another student wanted to have more productive arguments with her roommate (she didn't really want to stop arguing, she just wanted to get better at it), and the last, a professional translator, struggled with native speakers' elitism. By the time the instructor walked in to teach us empathy, we were all chummily commiserating about the ways other people made us crazy.

"Marshall Rosenberg taught that peace starts at home; verbal violence begins within our skins," the instructor said by way of introduction. Her name was Dian ("like Ian, with a D"), and she wore motorcycle boots and a snow-hat outfitted with a yarn mohawk. She carried a dulcimer along with her class materials just in case, she said, she felt like playing a gig later on. "He taught how to connect powerfully with ourselves. I believe in this so much, I wrote a song about it, called 'Love Yourself Harder.' And because I'm a New Yorker, I got a tattoo that says that too."

Dian wouldn't show us the tattoo, but she said if we had time, she might play us the song; she often incorporated music into her classes. We spent most of the evening, in fact, learning how to love ourselves harder—by way of identifying our own feelings when we listened to somebody else, and the ways these feelings linked to (perhaps unmet) needs. The idea is this: we can be blocked from truly hearing another person because our own feelings about their words or mode of expression take precedence. These feelings are usually linked to a need, so if we can first identify our own feeling, and then the need beneath it, and then possibly imagine a way to meet that need, we'll be open and clear to receive what the person is saying to us.

Whether or not empathy stems from mirror neurons, and

whether it should be understood as a skill or a moral orientation, there's still a *how* component to empathy, and this is it. NVC defines empathy fundamentally as a back-and-forth between the self and other: first identifying our own feelings and attendant needs so we can flow into another's, and then back again in an ongoing loop.

To practice, Dian had us all write down something somebody had said to us recently that was particularly triggering. My line came from my partner, Seth, during an argument: *You're too sensitive.* When Seth said it, I whisked right past the listening part and went in for the fight. I had answered, *Calling me sensitive is a way to deny responsibility for being a jerk.* If I had taken this class, I could have slowed down and taken an inventory of my feelings before rushing to speak. Dian passed out a sheet of paper with dozens of emotions listed on it, things like "apathetic," "mistrustful," "gloomy," "hesitant." For the "too sensitive" comment, I ticked off "depleted" and "lonely."

Then we turned to the "needs inventory" page—a more happy list of words. On this one, I checked "to matter." So, when Seth told me I was too sensitive, I felt depleted and lonely and needed to feel like I mattered. I realized this was the adult version of what school kids were learning in Roots of Empathy: slowing down to feel our feelings, label them, and connect them to needs to keep us from acting aggressively. If I had done this during my argument, I wouldn't have called Seth a jerk. The exercise was useful, sure, but I wasn't sure it was empathy.

The empathic part, Dian said, is when you practice the same process on your partner. First, you repeat their words back to them. As in, "I hear you saying I'm too sensitive." And then you guess what the need might be beneath the sentiment. In Seth's case, I would have said something like, "I'm guessing you might need a little more freedom to express yourself without concern about my reaction."

Our practiced responses sounded stiff, robotic, and nothing like real-life conversation. When Dian modeled empathic listening for us, she tweaked the language of the flight attendant's frustration.

"I hear you saying you're tired of passengers bossing you around; is that what you mean?"

Molly shook her head. "No. I'm sick of them not treating me like a person."

Dian didn't pause; she just looked into Molly's eyes and parroted her words exactly. "So you're sick of them not treating you like a person?"

"Yes!" Molly squealed, hopping happily in her seat. "You've got it exactly right!"

This seemed too simple, but it happened again and again: the more closely someone copied our words, the more satisfied—and yes, *understood*—we each felt. When Dian steered the conversation toward the need beneath Molly's feelings ("I'm guessing you want to have a little more choice internally about how you respond"), Molly was less sure; she wobbled her head into a questionable nod.

"My opinion, and I don't have the science to back this up, is that our cognitive function as a species developed faster than our emotional intelligence," Dian said. She had just cut her hand using the nutcracker on the walnuts and, not finding any ice in the Ayurvedic restaurant downstairs, she was nursing the wound with a bottle of cold salad dressing. "But human beings are naturally empathic."

Maybe it was because NVC, or Dian, subscribed to this hierarchy that we were applying cognitive tools to emotional experiences, but by the end of the night, I felt I had practiced repetition rather than learned to really listen with empathy, as I understood it. The flight attendant, the roommate, and the translator were strangers to me, and to actually grasp their stories, and to guess at the needs they were expressing, I would have needed more context, more time. Dian explained empathic communication as an infinity symbol, marking a figure eight in the air with her good hand: "What am I seeing, what are they seeing; what am I needing, what are they needing?"

This kind of back-and-forth, I thought, would work best in conflict-resolution settings. And in fact, NVC has been utilized in places like Rwanda, Israel, and Sierra Leone. But ultimately, the class provided a skill set, a method, a list of steps to take and things to say, and not an empathic force at work. We never defined empathy that night, or why we wanted it, and I felt more annoyed at Dian's drama with the salad dressing than compassionate toward her pain.

After handing out leaflets for her future talks, music gigs, and even her Airbnb, Dian asked us what we learned about empathy. We were eating minted couscous and spelt muffins from the restaurant downstairs. Between bites, Molly happily announced, "I learned about boundaries." I wondered if I learned anything about empathic listening; I hadn't heard one word about boundaries all night. Then again, I'm being concrete: Molly obviously listened to a subtext she alone was tuned to hear.

WHILE MAINSTREAM TRAINING GROUPS try to optimize empathy through our external actions, scientists are busy trying to first measure empathy internally and then prime the neuronal pumps for more. This measuring step is famously difficult, as empathy is only subjectively rendered through self-report—and its quantifiable outcomes (acts of generosity, statements of goodwill, buckets of tears) are third and fourth cousins to the birth of empathy itself. Even so, scientists are trying to pin empathy down: just who has it, who doesn't, and how can we gear the less empathic brains toward abundance?

Leo Moore is a graduate student in Dr. Marco Iacoboni's UCLA lab, and he is trying to do precisely this. He grew up in Oaxaca and wears flip-flops and button-down shirts with glitter polish on his nails "from like three days ago." So far, Moore has run seventy-eight brain scans on volunteers while they're doing now-classic low-level empathy exercises — things like imitating facial expressions or witnessing a disembodied hand get poked with a needle. He then asks these volunteers to do something that sounds entirely un-empathic: on a computer, alone in a room, the volunteers play the Dictator Game.

It isn't really a game, per se, but more of an economics or decision-theory experiment, first developed in 1982 and now replicated in well over a hundred publications. The basic premise is this: You (the Dictator) are given some kind of prize (usually money). You can either keep it all, give all of it away to another recipient, or share it in a ratio of your choosing. This recipient is entirely passive. The purported question is whether people are selfish or generous when they're allowed all the control.

"One of the problems with empathy is that there aren't a lot of behavioral outcomes for it," Leo explained, pushing a flop of curly brown hair from his forehead. To get to a measurable outcome, he first had to make a presumption: empathy drives prosocial behavior — like giving away money. This is a fairly big presumption but I went with it. Leo's hypothesis was that the more activation in the somatosensory areas there was in the pinpricked hand exercise, and the more there was emotional activation during the face mirroring, the more money they'd hand over in the Dictator Game.

What he found was more interesting. It turns out there's an area of the brain, the dorsolateral prefrontal cortex, that seems to actually *inhibit* empathy. (The left side appears to inhibit empathy for physical pain, the right side for emotional affect.) So, while Leo's volunteers' brains did light up as though their hands were actually being pricked, for instance, they were also activated in the region that controls, or modulates, pain response. The people with the more robust controls, or empathy inhibitors, gave the least away in the game.

In Moore's version of the game, after a volunteer has been scanned watching the pinpricks and facial expressions, she's brought to an empty room with a computer. She's told she will see photos and descriptions of twenty-four people, twelve of whom are real, twelve of whom do not exist. She will not know which is which. With each photo there are ten dollars at stake: the volunteer, or "dictator," can decide to give anywhere from zero to ten dollars and gets to keep the rest for herself. But here's the trick: the money will really be donated to twelve of the twenty-four computer people, but in only three out of the twenty-four cases is the money "real" for the dictator. In other words, the dictator stands to earn a total of thirty dollars—if she happens to give zero to the randomly marked three. The likelihood of this is slim: her only true chance at a full takeaway would be to give nothing to anybody.

"We know people tend to behave more in line with their reputation if they think they're being watched so we tell them, 'You can do whatever you want. Your data is anonymous. No one is ever going to know what you did,'" Leo explained, adding that this experiment also included no lying or deception. Research assistants never meet the volunteers, and they score data marked only by an ID number. "We almost encouraged subjects to be selfish."

I played the Dictator Game and, while my experience could have been skewed a bit because Leo was sitting nearby and I didn't stand to earn any real money, my results were smack in the realm of average. I sat at a computer screen and was told that all names and photos had been altered to protect confidentiality, and then a large face popped up on the screen, with text to the right. "This is Stella Lintz," it read. "She makes about $28,000 a year. Please make your offer." I was prompted to type a number between zero and ten and then the next face appeared. Each person wore the same neutral expression, and there were men and women, people of all races. I quickly discerned that the distinguishing factor was income; some of the people earned $15,000 or $30,000 per year; some earned upward of $200,000. I gave nothing to the ones in this upper echelon, everything to people who earned less than $30,000, and $5 or $6 to people in the middle, depending on whether I liked their eyes.

It turns out, Moore said, very few people gave away ten dollars each time to everybody, and very few people kept all the money for themselves. Most people were like me: they shared with the people who looked like they needed it and withheld from those who seemingly had plenty. But did they give more to people of the same race or gender? He didn't control for that; he just knew women were more generous than men, across the board.

"People who showed more activation in the control areas of their brain (inhibiting mirroring or empathizing) were less generous to the high-income players," Leo reported. In other words, these people contextualize more. Far from making them less empathic, this contextualizing ability is key to cognitive empathy. We need this kind of control and discernment to keep from merging emotionally with others and to be able to offer the kind of prosocial action Leo's experiment was designed to measure. "This is one in a million examples, but when you see a family member get really sad and you start to tear up yourself, at a certain point you go, 'Keep it together, I have to stay calm to help this person.'"

Moore proffered a truncated version of Hoffman's stages of empathic development. "I think the way development works is we start off with the affective empathy which you can barely call empathy . . . like when you're a baby, you cry because someone else cries. You don't have a distinct self-router," he said. "Then we develop these control systems that allow us to distinguish, 'That is them, this is me.'" For reasons we don't understand, some people develop stronger or weaker self/other barriers. Those diagnosed with schizophrenia, for example, struggle with recognizing what's generated inside and outside their own heads.

Leo recruited a few people with schizophrenia to play his Dictator Game. In the game, they gave away the same overall amount as the non-schizophrenic subjects, but they didn't modulate: they donated to rich and poor at random.

The most interesting part of this study was the most

Frankenstein-ish; it involved zapping subjects' brains with a magnetic field. Leo was looking to see if he could alter prosocial behavior by electrically altering the controls for empathy. With a magstim machine (the same device doctors employ for brain stimulation therapy in depression), Leo used magnets to send pulses through a subject's dorsolateral prefrontal cortex, temporarily tamping it down. For an hour or more, in the Dictator Game, the subject gave more money to the rich than he had before.

Getting shocked through the brain, at least at the low voltage used for transcranial magnetic stimulation, is more strange, or disquieting, than painful. In a room not much larger than a closet, Leo wiggled some knobs on a small monitor and then held a wand over the right side of my head. Two circles, hinged open like a jaw, met at the tip of the wand, and a magnetic pulse jumped between the coils and through my brain. It felt like a towel snapping in my skull. At that same instant, unbidden, my left arm jumped up spastically — a marionette arm, yanked by a string.

Leo laughed. "That was your motor region."

I wasn't laughing. Who was this guy in glitter polish, a person half my age wielding a wand that made people move and act in ways they couldn't control? In a flash, Leo morphed from fascinating scientist to bad wizard, but worse than that, my brain unlocked itself from the notion of being mine at all.

The deeply treasured Western notion of Self is a kind of dual self. This dual self harkens back to both Plato and Descartes, with a lot of religious ideology braiding itself in over the years. We tend to think that logic and reason and, for lack of a better word, functionality live in the brain, but our *real* selves, our soul selves, are immaterial and ineffable and perhaps exist beyond us when we die. This dual brain-soul self is united in an experiential "I," bounded by the borders of our physical body. And experiences like empathy — which draws on both cognition and something more soulful, like intuition — seem to be a bridge between the two.

The old doctor Hippocrates may have had it right when he determined that the brain was the basis for all feelings, thoughts, and ideas, but his contemporary Plato held the popular sway with his concept of a soul that existed before birth, inhabited a body, and left the body after death. Some 1,900 years later, Descartes famously theorized the roles of the brain and the soul, and the relationship between them. The brain, he said, responded to external stimuli like light and touch, and to commands from the soul—which was responsible for all mental functions like perceiving, thinking, hoping, deciding, and dreaming.

Today, we may logically know, and scientifically prove, that the brain in fact does think, perceive, dream, and decide, but the Cartesian shadow looms large. The duality is hard to shake: most of us have been trained to sense or believe that there's a "real self" (some call it a soul) outside the more pedestrian (if technically masterful) electrical workings of the brain. We simply can't believe that this Self, which can think its way into infinite elastic and expansive possibilities, is actually a corporeal mass of flesh inside a skull. That brain flesh just doesn't "feel" like all we are.

Until someone named Leo waves a wand and a silly magnet supplants an executive "real self" that should step up and override his shenanigans. I felt profoundly undignified, almost naked, when Leo hijacked my brain to move my arm.

Experientially, the brain seems to be what the ego, or self, directs. Leo's tricks reveal the reverse. The brain builds a self and the brain —bruised, shocked, drugged, or aged—can take that self away.

This can all seem pretty depressing, and in fact the relatively new field of neurophilosophy (basically the interface of philosophy's questions about choice, learning, and morality, with the gathering wisdom about the nervous system) largely busies itself with the ramifications of such discoveries. Patricia S. Churchland, who's taught neurophilosophy at the University of California, San Diego, writes that undergraduate students are drawn to neuroscience "as to a night bonfire in the woods" and yet are apprehensive about what their studies might conjure. They'll have to wrestle with the notion that there are neural correlates to states of consciousness, and invariably loosen their grip on the duality of a thinking brain and a feeling soul.

Churchland may be a hardcore materialist—and indeed she spends a good portion of one of her books explaining near-death experiences and spirit encounters as errant brain function—but as such, she asks important moral questions about intervening in what she calls the neuronal landscape of our selves. Adhering to the dual notion of brain and self probably helps justify mucking with the circuitry. We can alter things here and there, with drugs or magnets, because we believe there's a baseline to return to, some essential self that will emerge again when we stop our fiddling. It's a natural conclusion: so much of Western society hinges on personal responsibility, which in turn hinges on the belief in a cohesive, moral self, separate and distinct from the neuronal misfirings in an unwell brain. An Alzheimer's patient won't be punished for forgetting his pants; mentally ill patients can be unfit for trial and will never face the death penalty. But we are all a blur of our illness and wellness, of our synaptic maps and our unfortunate genes, and locating a discrete moral core untouched by these things is impossible because there isn't one. When we consider that this brain is everything we are, altering it intentionally takes on a much more serious tone.

I'm not saying that antidepressant drugs don't mitigate suffering, or that brain-based treatments couldn't be a viable alternative to life sentences for violent offenders. I am, however, questioning the specter of prosociality provoked by a couple of jolts to the cortex. In my lifetime, electroconvulsive therapy (ECT) has been utilized in this country on people like me to try to rid them of their socially objectionable behavior. As I write this, a landmark case in China exposed clinics trying to straighten the gays with electric shocks, so the treatment certainly hasn't gone away. Homosexuality, in certain circles, is still framed as an inherently selfish, and certainly deviant, orientation, and in that way it's made to sound eerily similar to the frame we place on people with empathy deficiencies. I worry about this view that a brain that alters its own notion of selfhood (with time, age, shock) is fundamentally mutable. It lends itself all too easily to experiments designed to fix the irregular, and all around the world, the irregular is me. In the laboratory scenario, empathy is posited as a set of modifiable behaviors. The laboratory itself is positioned in a society where empathy is less an idea or even an inquiry than a set of skills and tools. From all directions, empathy is an act, rather than a way, and acts are always subject to social control. It's a snake eating its tail: change the acts by changing the brain, which by definition changes the person, who then understands the acts anew and wants to change them up again. There's no moral center to this story.

THE MOST EXTREME, and yet logical, implication of this thought experiment is its real-world application to psychopaths. So many discussions about empathy veer into psychopathology because that's the diagnosis where empathy has not faltered but rather skipped its entrance altogether. And psychopaths, we've decided, are simply not treatable with any form of traditional psychotherapy. Aside from exhibiting a lack of empathy, psychopaths also generally lie, have little to no remorse or guilt, are manipulative, and lack long-term goals—all the while carrying a grandiose sense of self-worth. They don't make very good patients. But they could, some doctors think, respond to other kinds of treatments. And maybe if we could begin to understand the brains of people where empathy isn't, we might just get a hook into what empathy *is*.

Interestingly, even though the root of the word means *soul* (psycho) *suffering* (-pathy), we seem to have little empathy for those without it. Kent Kiehl, Ph.D., is hailed as one of the world's experts on psychopaths, particularly on their neurobiology, and is the author of *The Psychopath Whisperer: The Science of Those Without a Conscience*. Kiehl says that socially, we've poured far fewer resources into researching alternative cures to psychopathy than we have to, say, schizophrenia. Schizophrenics are considered victims, while psychopaths are perpetrators.

"If we were to dedicate half the resources to treating psychopathy that we do to treating cancer, our prisons would be one third the size they are today," Kiehl told me over the phone from his office in New Mexico. In fact, it's primarily inside the criminal justice system that the term "psychopath" even comes up. Medically, psychopathology is not an actual identification; no psychiatric or psychological association has sanctioned an official diagnosis. Psychopathy is both a long and historically debated list of qualifying features that's now labeled broadly in the Diagnostic and Statistical Manual of Mental Disorders (DSM) as "antisocial personality disorder"—characterized by antisocial and disinhibited behavior, and diminished empathy and remorse. Maybe it's this lack of a clinical designation (muddied further by the cousin term, "sociopathy," which is thought to be less biological in origin and whose sufferers exhibit many of the same traits, though sometimes in less severe form) that fosters a diminished financial interest. Or maybe it's because people think psychopaths end up in prison anyway—experts estimate that 1 percent of the general population is psychopathic, as opposed to upward of 20 percent of the prison population. There certainly aren't the same family support groups lobbying for their cure the way there are for other kinds of patients who score low on empathy affect, like people with schizophrenia, autism, or ADHD.

But it's precisely because psychopaths commit crimes that Kiehl wants to understand the ways their brains work: crime, he says, has a trillion-dollar price tag in this country, not to mention the collective psychic and emotional toll this crime carries. And a psychopath is between four and eight times more likely to recommit than your average criminal—and to do so violently. If we could just understand this fifth of the current 1.5 million state and federal prison inmates, we would all be better off.

In 2007, Kiehl began wheeling a portable fMRI machine behind the gates of Western New Mexico Correctional Facility, and to date he has scanned more than five hundred criminal psychopaths and three thousand other offenders at multiple sites. To "count" as a psychopath, inmates had to score between thirty and the maximum forty on the diagnostic gold standard, the Hare Psychopathy Checklist-Revised (an average score for an average male is four). Developed and published by a man named Robert Hare in 1991, the checklist picks up where the DSM leaves off. Kiehl estimates that twice as many people will qualify for antisocial personality disorder as for pure psychopathy. Psychologists and forensics experts use the checklist as the singular, reliable measure to indicate a true psychopath: it's composed of a semi-structured interview and a comprehensive file review that includes police reports, social worker assessments, family and employment history, and so on. Even if he hadn't sorted through all of this material, Kiehl writes that he can often sense, instinctively, who is and isn't a psychopath; after hundreds of interviews, he has enough practice. Psychopaths can be exceedingly charming, talkative, funny—but there's simply something "off" about the person. Like empathy itself, experiencing psychopathology is a sort of singular, gut-level thing. It's hard to describe, but you know it when you feel it.

When I met a person I believed to be a psychopath, I felt the tiniest chill in my belly, but I pushed it down. Caroline (not her real name) was just a teenager, and in so many ways just like the dozens of other teenagers I've interviewed for books and articles about foster kids and street kids. I met Caroline through a friend of a friend; we talked a couple of times about her past experiences and her future plans, which, like most kids I knew, didn't extend beyond a couple of months. Caroline wanted money, and she wanted revenge against some other girls for perceived slights. And here was the difference:

lots of kids I knew said they were "gonna kill that bitch," but with Caroline, I couldn't feel the soft underbelly of fear or shame or loss beneath the bravado. I couldn't feel anything at all except the chill.

I've worked on and off for ten years teaching in a women's prison, and I never met someone quite like Caroline. I've met murderers that I thought I understood; they told me stories of battering boyfriends or of drugs, and, yes, maybe they were feeding me lines, but there was also that indisputable ping of connection. Caroline was funnier than most inmates I've taught; she wore fashionable clothes and went clubbing every weekend with whatever boyfriend of the week she fancied. She had been in some trouble for stealing and fighting, but superficially, she seemed normal enough for a kid who came from the streets. I certainly didn't give Caroline the Hare Checklist, but when she said the line about the killing, I knew, in a flash and in a way I've never felt before or since, that she could kill me too.

ON THE PHONE, Kiehl sounds younger than his actual middle age and his voice carries an edge of impatience. His primary work is to translate his hundreds of scans into evidence of psychopathology's biological deviance from the so-called norm, and to use that to target and develop treatment. In his book, Kiehl describes an imaging study of 256 male offenders, and detecting atrophy, or reduced grey matter, in the paralimbic systems of those correlated with psychopathy. It's a significant finding, but it's also just a start—the paralimbic system encompasses the orbital frontal cortex, the amygdala, the hippocampus, the insula, the temporal pole, and the interior and posterior cingulate—a considerable chunk of neural real estate to begin targeting treatment. Kiehl is also quick to note that the discovery isn't causal; in other words, we don't know whether the abnormalities were inborn and caused the psychopathic behavior, or whether the behavior led to structural changes in the brain.

Kiehl does have a few clues, however, that point toward the inborn theory. One is that the psychopaths he's interviewed in prison come from deeply varied backgrounds; some grew up in loving families, some were abused or neglected as children; they're rich, they're poor, they're in between. The second clue is that he's started scanning teenage offenders. These younger brains, ostensibly, wouldn't have clocked enough years to show such drastic atrophy if there hadn't been some aberrance to begin with.

Kiehl processed the brain scans of two hundred teenage boys from a maximum-security juvenile prison, most of whom had been convicted of multiple felonies. Even in criminal settings, we don't grant people the official label of psychopath until they're adults; children are handed a broader catch-all category called "callous and unemotional traits," as determined by a Youth Psychopathy Checklist. Kiehl ran this checklist by all of his subjects, and the callous and unemotional kids had precisely the same paralimbic brain abnormalities as their adult psychopathic counterparts.

In a kind of mainstream cultural imagination, the adult criminal psychopath was once a kid who wet his bed, hurt animals, and lit things on fire. This cluster of behaviors is called the Mac-Donald Triad, and in fact many adult murderers do exhibit the triad as kids. But the formula doesn't go the other direction; the vast majority of bed-wetting, fire-hungry, and even sadistic children will not go on to commit heinous crimes. Predictive labeling can be dangerous. Kiehl talks about a boy he knows who was socially isolated and subject to delusions and hence entirely suggestible. When a doctor erroneously called him a psychopath, the teenager wanted to fulfill the prophecy and stabbed a stranger in her home.

This is an extreme example, but it reflects the fear that parents, doctors, and specialists carry about stigmatizing children with a terrifying title. It's why we give them the softer-sounding "traits"— even if, as Kiehl's research suggests, some kids are born with a true disability.

"I think you have to make a choice: either you believe in prediction or you don't," Kiehl said. "But the fact is we are making predictions all the time. Judges are predicting when they decide to put someone on parole, put them away for life, send them home with an ankle bracelet. I think we should be helping them make these predictions with the best science—and the brain is the ground truth."

Kiehl admits that the scanning science isn't adequate to make full-scale predictions yet, but he assumes it will be in the future, and to reserve such predictions only for the adult courtroom is also to withhold potentially life-saving youth treatment. For example, with the bed-wetters: only 15 percent will continue past the age of five, and those kids have developmental delays or abnormalities in one of four or more neural pathways. One of these pathways leads through the amygdala—the brain region responsible for recognizing fearful faces, something psychopaths can't do. Kiehl's theory is that the amygdala circuit kids (who also light fires and hurt animals) could be the ones to commit heinous crimes down the line.

If we could narrow down the MacDonald Triad to a more clinically predictive subgroup, what would we do with them? After all, Kiehl claims, "the circuit for the real emotional experience of empathy doesn't engage in psychopaths." Still, in children, Kiehl likens the empathy to a weakened muscle: "You have to develop crutches that can make it stronger."

In Australia, the director of the Child Behavior Research Clinic at the University of New South Wales, Mark R. Dadds, is trying experimental therapies on callous and unemotional children as young as six. Because of the amygdala dysfunction, these kids don't recognize fear in others' faces, which Dadds says is critical to recognizing that people, or animals, are sentient beings. Knowing, and then caring, that another person is afraid is what stops you from hurting them. In other words: empathy. But knowing how to see the fear is the first part.

So Dadds is focusing on the eyes. Callous/unemotional kids interpreted fearful faces as "neutral" or "disgusted"—but it turns out, they weren't looking where most of us do, into the subjects' eyes. When these same kids were directed to look at the eyes, they guessed correctly, and saw fear. Further studies need to be done, but this could be one big hint: if we can train children with indications of future psychopathology to habitually look toward the eyes, we may help them to understand what others are feeling and to empathize, even if it doesn't come naturally.

This training, Dadds believes, is not only useful for the way a child treats others but for the way others treat him. In another study, callous/unemotional kids didn't return their mother's gaze when she told them she loved them. This lack of eye contact could have a snowball effect: when parents don't feel reciprocal emotions through the eyes of their child, they grow more frustrated; the child gets stressed and ultimately aggressive, so the parents provide less positive, loving feedback, and the cycle continues until the failure to gaze can become, Dadds hypothesizes, "cascading errors affecting the development of empathy and social functioning."

Caroline, the teenager I believe was a psychopath, met my eyes, but she didn't lock in. It was subtle, the experience of Caroline's gaze, but powerful too — it seemed she was looking at my eyes but not into them. I couldn't feel myself reflected.

Even as I write this, though, I hesitate. I recognize that eye gaze can be cultural, individual, that my expectations for reciprocity are based on my own socially derived experiences with it. Judging Caroline is akin to judging my students for their learning styles in the classroom, which I try so hard not to do. I've had students from all parts of the world, students who make exacting eye contact as a challenge and students who avert their eyes out of deference, students with Asperger's, and students so glued to their phones that merely looking up has become a sort of deviance. I remind myself that my interpretations of student expressions and behavior are frequently wrong, simply because I don't know their context.

My gut feeling about someone, that chill I felt with Caroline, is both the key to my empathy and its impediment. Caroline told me she never once felt afraid, and in her eyes I felt an intelligent cruelty laced through a flat kind of tedium. Feeling all that was a kind of empathy. But in order to feel *for* Caroline, I'd have to overcome what I was seeing. I'd have to buck my own fear to imagine her life without it.

Christian Keysers, a neuroscientist in the Netherlands who studies empathy, says that even criminal psychopaths have this ability to switch on the empathy—it's just not their default position. In an fMRI scanner, Keysers and his lab showed psychopathic Dutch inmates images of hands interacting in neutral, loving, socially rejecting, or physically painful ways. In the control group, men's brains were vicariously activated by the images, as though they were experiencing the gestures themselves. The psychopaths, predictably, showed no such empathic activation. However, when they were told expressly to empathize with the hands they were seeing, their brains lit up, just like the control group. It's not that psychopaths can't empathize; it's that they don't.

But combine this propensity for empathy with early eye-gaze training and controlled carrot-stick behavior modification (Kiehl says a system of graduated rewards and punishments at a youth correctional facility is working well on the callous/unemotional kids there), and we may have the scaffolding for teaching empathy to the heretofore supposedly unteachable.

All of this shows that training in empathy requires practicing its first lesson, seeing through the eyes of the other. Psychopaths are known to think in terms of short-term gain, not long-term goals; it's the reason the slower, nuanced psychotherapy hasn't worked. Any treatment has to use this as a frame (look in the eyes and you'll get some tangible reward) until, perhaps, the experience becomes its own prize or the brain has rewired itself significantly, or both.

I don't know if these approaches lean toward cures, or even staying power, but I applaud the investigative work. For me, with Caroline, I unfortunately found that self-preservation trumped the empathic impulse. As soon as I could sense that I was feeling her but she wasn't feeling me, I only wanted to get away. And in this I may be siding with the majority who shunt psychopathy research to the sidelines. I was afraid of her. Fear is what forms a root of recognizing the other as human, a building block of empathy, and it's what psychopaths don't feel. Yet fear also forecloses the possibility of understanding and building a kind of moral imagination about the other; it's our hope and hindrance at once.

4

Ars Empathia

One cold winter afternoon, I was taking a cab to appear on a public radio show for authors. We were tasked with the topic "Books That Changed Our Minds." Of course, every book changes our mind in some way, and in fact, just a few months before that cab ride, a whole host of articles lauded two new studies that showed reading literary fiction boosted empathy.

During the ride, the driver, Umar, asked me what I did for a living (at first, because of my glasses, he presumed I was in IT). I told him I was a writer, and he said he was too.

"The minute you become a cabbie, you also become a writer," Umar said. I asked him why.

"Because you learn about another's perspective and you always have movement," he answered. "That's what a story is."

Umar was more succinct than I am, but that's essentially what I teach in my writing classes: perspective and movement. Usually, the two are intertwined. A changing perspective induces a (psychological or physical) movement, and vice versa. This is also why we read.

One of the literary empathy studies was designed by social psychologists at the New School in New York, and it showed that after reading literary fiction for three to five minutes (as opposed to popular fiction or science writing), subjects were more likely to immediately decipher the emotions in photographs of eyes or full faces. The other study, out of the Netherlands, tracked empathy over a longer stretch of time. Dutch students were asked to read either a Sherlock Holmes story or a chapter from José Saramago's *Blindness* for an entire week. A control group read newspaper articles. When both groups self-reported their levels of empathy, the fiction group scored higher both immediately after the experiment and one week later.

I have a couple of reactions to studies like these. The first is to question their impetus. At a time when both funding and collective interest in art are on the brink, data that point to art's measurable usefulness can rally supporters to the cause. (Authors of the New School study cite the adoption of the Common Core, which calls for less emphasis on literature in high school, in secondary schools in forty-six states.) This could be, ostensibly, fine, except that art by nature is experiential, the stuff of thought and feeling. Reducing literature to quantifiable outcomes is to limit our understanding of its reach and meaning, and potentially its production. In general, most of us don't read solely because it's going to give us something or do something for us; that's far too narrow a goal. We read for pleasure, for escape, for possibility; we read because we don't know what we're going to get. And we do get different things from different books: aesthetic ideas, new emotional pliability, imaginative flights, and so on. But if empathy is the objective-du-jour, and we start reading (or writing) books with this in mind, we miss the sea we're swimming in. Hyper-goal-oriented art isn't art; it's propaganda.

THAT SAID, EMPATHY is so inherent to reading, the studies also made me laugh a little. It was as though scientists proved that trees gave shade. Books are one way we imagine other lives; we can inhabit, for a moment, the mind of a psychopath or an adulterer or a nun, when we might never be those things ourselves.

While both studies focused on reading, movies and plays and paintings, sculpture and dance, also invoke empathy. We look to them for the transport. That linkage between empathy and artistic experience is baked into the history of the term itself. After all, the philosopher Robert Vischer—the first person to use the word *Einfühlung,* "feeling into," before Theodor Lipps published on it extensively—came of age during intense debates about aesthetics in art. During the early and mid-nineteenth century, these debates centered on the most pleasing shapes and an attempt to locate a science of forms based on the golden rectangle. But then the Romantics came along and found these discussions arid and empty; they argued for art's inherent feeling and emotion. Vischer was a part of this time. He said we appreciate art because we feel our way into it; *Einfühlung* was later extended as a theory to explain the way we come to know others' minds. Rather than intellectually deducing someone's state of mind through observation (I see a frown, he must be angry), *Einfühlung*/empathy posits that we see a frown, feel that frown inside ourselves, know the emotions attached to frowning, and thereby understand the experience of the other. This is immediate and instinctive.

The ways we intuit or interpret another's mental state is its own field of study for both philosophers and cognitive psychologists—it's called "Theory of Mind" (ToM). We've been thinking about ToM long before Lipps and Vischer and long before we called it ToM; René Descartes's "I think therefore I am" set a broad stage for standing outside a mind and peering in. Today, people argue over whether animals have a theory of mind and whether preverbal children can understand a parent's intention if different from their own. By the age of four, we know, most children can pass a basic "false belief" test. This means if they watch a video of Charlie placing his chocolate on the shelf and then leaving the room only to have his mother come in and take the chocolate away, they'll discern that Charlie won't know where his candy went when he comes looking for it later. In other words, they can have a theory about Charlie's mind.

ToM is a base note for empathy; you have to know that someone's beliefs, knowledge, or feelings are separate from yours in order to empathize with them. It's also critical for understanding stories. In the New School study, participants who read literary fiction scored higher on ToM tests than those who read popular fiction because, the authors posit, popular fiction "tends to portray the world and characters as internally consistent and predictable." Readers don't need to emotionally stretch to understand a character's motivations. Literary fiction, by contrast, "uniquely engages the psychological processes needed to gain access to characters' subjective experiences." We build fully fleshed-out people from the thin stuff of words; we imagine them before and after the curtain falls on their scenes; we ascribe motivation to gestures and glances.

I have a friend who's a historical novelist; her work requires readers to enter the mindscapes of characters who live in completely unfamiliar material worlds. When I first told her I was working on a nonfiction book about empathy and asked her what she thought, her answer surprised me.

"I feel threatened," she said. "Empathy is what novelists do."

It was as though exploring a car's engine could diminish the ride, at least in my friend's mind. Or else she thought, as the literature studies indicated, that fiction has the corner on empathy. But for me, it's not just the finely wrought or expressively complex fictional characters that trigger a ToM response; literary nonfiction can also elevate readers into worlds outside their own and take some kind of moral inventory. Sometimes, with attentive reading, we project ourselves into the mind of the author creating those concepts on the page; that forces a kind of empathy, too. Often, you can feel the act of the writing, the struggle or the discovery. Susan Sontag expressed it well, claiming, "Writing is an embrace, a being embraced: every idea is an idea reaching out."

On the radio show where I had to pick one book that changed my mind, I ultimately chose nonfiction. James Baldwin is an author whose essays change my mind every time I read them, and that day I talked about *Notes of a Native Son*. I've read the title essay in that book over a dozen times because I teach it so often, and because the ending is near-perfect. In the piece, Baldwin is searching to understand his father, whom he hated and who hated the world, only to discover that his father's bitterness was inherent to living in the world and that it's a bitterness that Baldwin inherited. We feel empathy for everyone here, for the character Baldwin has written himself to be, but also for the author behind the words, the human being he is struggling to become. Baldwin's ending, that "one would have to hold in the mind forever two ideas which seemed to be in opposition," is a paradox, as is its solution. One idea is to accept, without rancor, injustice. The other is to fight that injustice with all one's strength. While these seemingly oppositional ideas are in the mind, the fight begins in the heart, and, he writes, "it had now been laid to my charge to keep my own heart free of hatred and despair."

I've thought about this interplay between the head and the heart many times; it's one metaphor for empathy. When the connection is severed—as when Baldwin feels the "click" at the nape of his neck just before he assaults a racist waitress "as though some interior string connecting my head to my body had been cut"—empathy stops. I've thought about this intellectual task of emotional work, of freeing the heart of hatred, and because I *feel* for Baldwin, I *think* perhaps I can do it too. That is the empathy of good nonfiction, or of art.

This book enters the world at a time when the black body, particularly the black male body, is the site of radical injustice. It always has been, of course, but the lens has widened to capture endemic police violence for a national and increasingly motivated audience. My own rage and despair are heightened as I march with the other protesters in the Black Lives Matter actions and think of the riots in Baldwin's *Notes,* and I know that the body cameras or commissioner reviews on offer are but bandages for the systemic poison that Baldwin describes and which is in us still. And I think of the way that I fight when I am most hurt and hopeless, which is not with compassion but with the rage of a wounded animal lashing out. Which is to say, it's precisely when you want to blame the other — the police, our genocidal forefathers, the ignorant neighbor — that it's hardest to find the softness within.

While I wrote this book, my partner of ten years was shifting from being perceived as a female body to being perceived as a male body. I could write that Seth is transgender and transitioned from female to male but that wouldn't be accurate to his lived experience. The truth is he never felt like one or the other, but some years ago he had top surgery and in 2014, he started taking testosterone in the hopes of easing the dysphoria he had always felt. People on the streets, in shops, at the gym, started treating him as a man, and by that I mean they not only called him "sir" but angled with him for talking space, shot competitive gazes, or flirted, depending on their gender and social position. For Seth, his interior world was constant but the outside cues had flipped. And then, maybe because the outside affects the inside, or maybe because of the hormones, Seth's feelings, his emotionality, changed too. Seth grew facial hair and a deeper voice, but he also developed a new need for solitude and a quicker temper. And then we began to fight.

I had always believed myself empathic to Seth's transition: I have a transgender foster daughter; I've written two books on trans issues; I'm deeply connected with and in this community. And yet when we started arguing more and I felt like my relationship was threatened, I lost my tenuous hold on a Baldwin paradox. I got bitter. How could Seth, who was a feminist, who had been socialized female, be slipping into stereotyped behaviors? I blamed outside things: the hormones, the idea of hormones, the pressure or perhaps the allure of some kind of psychological conformity with a male prototype, anything to avoid listening to Seth, who was saying he was retreating and angry because I was the one who was fighting all the time. It wasn't true. He was the one who had changed. We had both fought against the injustice of the artificial male/female binary, and he had brought the binary roaring into our home. I didn't see the ways his old bitterness was now mine to bear.

Sometime after the fighting began, Seth and I went to see a play at the Brooklyn Academy of Music that was based on a book I'd been teaching in my classes for years. Called *A Human Being Died That Night,* it's the true story of a black South African psychologist named Dr. Pumla Gobodo-Madikizela, who interviews the white former chief of Vlakplaas, apartheid's death squad. His real name is Eugene de Kock, but he's known as Prime Evil.

The action of the play revolves around de Kock's various disclosures, but the point of the play is Gobodo-Madikizela's own empathy. She must decide whether she can understand and then forgive him.

Theater, like literature, has also been studied for its effects on empathy. Schoolchildren who attend live theater (as opposed to watching a televised version or reading a script) are better able to interpret the emotional affect in photographs of human eyes. Dance, as well, is subject to this scrutiny, as researchers study kinesthetic empathy, or the ways we feel others' movement in our bodies. Music too (either listening or playing) bumps the empathic response. Empathy happens to be the lens we like right now, but I imagine if the measurement were self-esteem or generosity or curiosity, researchers could show appreciable increases in these realms too. The bottom line is, the arts are good for you. But with theater specifically, the actors are generally trained to embody or empathize with other people, their characters. We gauge the actors' success by how accurately they do this, or how acutely we feel their emotions and experiences in ourselves. Live theater is exciting because the actors are then pulling from the feeling of the crowd. It's an empathy loop all around.

The theater in Brooklyn was packed. Some South Africans, but mostly Americans. How far from our experience were the death squads, apartheid, a prison cell in Pretoria? The whole play is staged from this one cell, Gobodo-Madikizela and de Kock, in his orange jumpsuit, sitting across a table from each other, de Kock shackled to his chair. Their talk is intimate, though de Kock takes up most of the space, at first hedging the psychoanalyst's questions with out-landish stories, and then finally softening into confession. At one point, Gobodo-Madikizela is moved by de Kock's story of the boy he once was, overpowered by a brutish father, commandeered by a sick regime, and she reaches across the table and touches his hand. Later, de Kock tells her, "That was my trigger hand you touched."

The audience collectively gasped. We might not have lived through apartheid in the townships the way Gobodo-Madikizela had, or met a man who had personally killed or tortured people, but we had all reached out to someone in kindness and been stung. We all entered the play right there.

Multiple studies show, especially in relation to charitable giving, that people respond more readily to one person's individual need than to a story of mass atrocity. Perhaps the sadness doesn't stretch, or our psyches put up blocks when the numbers are too big, or the numbers become abstractions, or all three. But theater pinpoints, crystallizes, a singular person's experience within the collective weight of his con-text. Part of de Kock's message in the play is to say that he was one of many monsters, a sick cog in the very sick machine that was apart-heid. Most of these monsters weren't behind bars; some gave direct orders, and some simply benefited from the regime and did nothing. In other words, to live in that country meant to touch many trigger hands. And yet. Gobodo-Madikizela had to contend with that one, singular statement, from one, singular person, and decide: was he a sadist, reveling in her discomfort, or was he divulging his sin before her, as one broken man hoping to be fully seen? At some point, in the darkness, I reached over the armrest and held Seth's hand, knowing we, like the rest of the audience, were struggling with this question, but mostly grateful for our connection.

· · ·

I've always been interested in art that's both empathic toward and critical of its subject matter because it seems to be the most difficult and full of possibility. Pure critique is just a rant without ears, and art that's too sympathetic becomes sentimental or just mere representation. But visual, performance, musical, or literary art that can both stand inside its subject as the subject itself would stand, and then also cast a new ground for that standing — that to me proffers a kind of hope. Like *A Human Being Died That Night* or like Baldwin's work, this kind of art breaks down the binary of us and them while not softening into a kind of humanistic or relativist "we're all the same" refrain.

Artistic empathy, to me, isn't a mimetic exchange but rather a chance to deeply see, and to dispute, the constructs around us — without losing that original sight. I admire artists who engender both compassion and a challenge. When that balance is right, their work can offer chances, or pathways, through the seemingly intractable battles that roar everywhere else.

I spent a long time talking with one artist who walks this line of artistic empathy particularly well. Her name is Amber Hawk Swanson, and she's obviously one of thousands I could have interviewed, but she struck my interest because she does feminist performance art and befriends the subjects of her critical gaze. I came of age, and came out, at the end of the 1980s and early 1990s, when second-wave feminism was waning and the third wave was breaking through — a time when performance artists like Annie Sprinkle, Karen Finley, and the Guerrilla Girls were carving a path for artists like Hawk Swanson. It was the time of ACT UP, the Meese Commission Report, and the National Endowment for the Arts' defunding of cutting-edge artists, when artists could be really angry — and also pro-joy, pro-pleasure, pro-sex. These artists challenged the systems of oppression all around them while at the same time deeply empathized with the disenfranchised or dispossessed. Their work said, Welcome, have some fun. Hawk Swanson's art speaks back to this tradition but goes further: it attempts not only to engender empathy toward both the oppressed and the oppressor but to scramble this binary altogether.

Amber works with Real Dolls, the expensive, realistic silicone sex dolls that made their mainstream debut in the 2007 movie *Lars and the Real Girl.* At first blush, Amber's work seems confrontational, a feminist critique of a culture that treats women as pliable, usable objects. She has brought her doll to highly ritualized, hyper-gendered spaces like tailgate parties and beauty pageants and filmed the results. (Within minutes of spotting the Real Doll perched on a lawn chair in the parking lot at a crowded football game, five men were upon her, their flies open, publicly violating the doll's every available orifice.) But Amber's doll isn't just one of the eight sexy prototypes the manufacturers had on offer when she had hers constructed; her face is a precise replica of Amber's own at twenty-six. Amber married this doll in a staged ceremony and lived with her for a year. Later, once Amber Doll had been terribly marred and damaged through her various public performances, Amber cut her up and turned her into a sculpture of Tilikum, the Sea World orca famous for killing its captors.

"I'm interested in captivity in multiple levels," Hawk Swanson said to me, describing her own complicity in feminine constructions. She is six feet tall and high-femme: she has long black hair and a creamy complexion, and she's usually wearing wedge sandals and a clingy wrap dress from the 1970s; for one of her performances she wore a pistachio pantsuit with red kitten heels.

But Amber's also interested in the men who have relationships with real dolls, often called Doll Husbands. Early in her project, Amber started meeting these men, going to their conventions, listening to their reasons for buying the dolls, understanding their love. Generating empathy. I thought that these guys would hate Amber's work; she cut up her doll and turned it into a whale. But they didn't. They participated in it.

"We were having brunch at this diner after DolLApalooza, and I made a joke that they should donate their retired dolls to the whale reclamation center," Amber said. DolLApalooza is one of the two annual meetups for doll owners and takes place in the doll factories in southern California; the second is at a hunting lodge in Pennsylvania. At the time she didn't take her own comment seriously; she had finished with the Tilikum project and wasn't interested in building any more whales. But then one of the more prominent and well-known spokespeople for the doll community spoke up and offered to donate his silicone wife's body to the whale reclamation center, and the "Lolita Project" was born.

That person was Davecat, and he's been the subject of several documentaries and news clips. Davecat calls himself an iDollator and a technosexual, and has claimed in many interviews that synthetic relationships work better for him because synthetics won't lie, cheat, change their personalities, or leave him for somebody else. Davecat bought his first doll, Sidore, in 2000; they wear matching wedding bands that say "Synthetik [*sic*] love lasts forever." Davecat has since purchased a second synthetic, Elena, who's his mistress and friend to Sidore while he's at work.

To interviewers' inevitable questions about whether he's objectifying women through his dolls, Davecat claims the opposite: he says that he's personifying objects. He says men who objectify women would have been doing so before learning about synthetics, and most iDollators treat their dolls with tremendous care and kindness. The doll bodies usually weigh somewhere around seventy-five pounds, with silicone skin, removable wigs and tongues, and a posable PVC skeleton. Davecat likes to dress both Elena and Sidore up for photo shoots, stay in and watch videos or go online with them (both dolls have Twitter accounts), and move them around his one-bedroom apartment. Such activity invariably wears down the doll, and Sidore has been through three bodies, though she's kept her head. Her second body went to Amber.

"I'm obsessed with the fact that there's a killer whale named Lo-lita," Amber said to me from her studio in Brooklyn, describing the orca who's lived for over forty-five years in a sixty-by-eighty-foot tank at the Miami Seaquarium. "I'm pretty obsessed in general with a captive body being labeled as seductive as a way to erase its status as captive, and I knew that this act could address that obsession."

The "act" was a six-day, seventy-hour performance, livestreamed for 45,000 viewers. Wearing a white frilly apron and saddle shoes, Amber dismembers two full-bodied dolls with saws and X-Acto blades—one is Sidore, and the other is Heather, donated by a man named Jesse. Next to Amber, Davecat is perched on a stool, dressed in grey slacks and a tie, reading the entire *Lolita* manuscript. The effect is mesmerizing.

"There's really nothing wrong with being moved to distraction by girl children," Davecat reads as Amber stacks arms and legs, feet and fingers, in preparation for their reincarnation as Lolita. The actual Lolita used to share her tank with a killer whale named Hugo, who died of a brain aneurysm caused by repeatedly smashing his head against the concrete walls of his confinement. For years, activists have argued for Lolita's release, claiming that the sound waves bouncing off the tank and the limited mobility (orcas generally swim hundreds of miles per day) cause profound suffering. Via a live feed, Amber interviews marine mammal specialists about this suffering as she begins to bolt and staple and stitch a whale from the bits of human (silicone) form. A camera inside Seaquarium films Lolita performing her stage show, as Amber applies black and white paint to the sculpture.

Amber is tender, almost loving, as she works with the silicone, and this tenderness is reflected in a story from Jesse, the owner of Heather, whose body is also being incorporated into Lolita.

"The allure of [dolls] is that you're taking care of someone," Jesse says. His voice is disembodied; he's talking via speakerphone to Amber and Davecat as they meticulously clean the silicone. Now Jesse has a new doll, named Rhiannon. "When my wife was in bed with cancer, all I really wanted was for her to look to me for help . . . That's why I have Rhiannon to bathe or dress or clothe or fix her hair or whatever, I'm feeling the same thing I felt when I was taking care of my wife."

I asked Amber if she viewed dolls as captive bodies, and she said no, though she acknowledged that the theme is there. This idea, however, is "complicated by the participation of the doll owners themselves," who present a much more nuanced picture of the captor/captive dichotomy. Back in 2005, when Amber was first reading about doll husbands, these men were usually typecast as misogynist outsiders. Amber said the descriptions were personal and mean. People on feminist sites were calling doll owners "fat, ugly people who can't get dates" (the very slurs used against feminists), and Amber was intrigued to get to know the people behind the stereotypes. Sexual violence, and violation, are other themes that people see in both the dolls and in Amber's work, but she's interested in "pulling the violent space apart to see the tenderness that exists within it."

Amber calls herself a "material translator" between the art community and the doll community, and I admit, before I saw her work, I needed such interpretation. When I first heard about them, I had written off Real Dolls as mere sex toys and their buyers as likely relationally deficient in some profound way. Jesse, the doll owner whose wife died of cancer, was my route to understanding. In another performance piece, called "Doll Closet," Jesse is again on speakerphone. For fifteen years, Jesse kept his old doll Heather in a room with a sealed-off closet space, for which Jesse constructed a secret door with hinges on the inside — a kind of panic room. His wife never knew about the closet. Jesse now has a new wife, and Rhiannon now has a space outside the home.

"I'm trying to be more of a man, to live up to the expectations of a man," Jesse says. His accent has a slight southern lilt. But he "likes soft things, likes fancy things." He likes to dress in women's clothes.

Once, when he was just driving around in a mini skirt and heels, he was pulled over by the cops. They detained him for twenty minutes and then told him his friends wouldn't like to know what he was up to and ordered him home to get changed. He's now had his women's clothes and shoes altered to fit Rhiannon; he projects all his fantasies onto her. "It's probably better for me to keep it in the closet than to be ridiculed. It's one of the reasons a lot of guys like me have dolls."

My heart cracked open when I heard this. I've known so many people like Jesse, barred by their community or family or their own internalized stigma from expressing themselves, and they find a surrogate outlet. For Seth, the outlet was sports; he became a disciplined and intense athlete in an attempt to mold his musculature away from the feminine. It didn't work — the gender dysphoria chewed at him daily — but he, like Jesse, tried to keep it all hidden and contained. He thought he should learn to be satisfied with the body he was born with. One of our first arguments was about babies. Seth said that no baby is born hating its body; they learn that through gendered cultural norms. He wanted perhaps to get back to that pre-hating state, but I argued that he lived in the world and should express himself fully, as a reconfigured body, within it.

Amber's work explores what's possible in the hidden, cut-off spaces, what's possible in the closet. In "Doll Closet," Amber reconstructs Jesse's closet out of plywood and the same locking-pin system, as he calls in with instructions and guidance. All of this is livestreamed over several days with viewers posting their thoughts. In this way, what was once private becomes public. This is like the transgender or gender-variant body itself, I think, as a body that was once held safely only in the imagination becomes a site for public scrutiny and commentary. The closet, too, has always been a place for both queer repression and connection. When I was young and just coming out, for instance, I was forced into the closet by my family for a bit but I knew I wasn't alone there. I knew there were others too, hidden away, and that assembly brought solace.

Today, the internet serves as a kind of closet where queers of all kinds can both find one another and remain safely anonymous. Most of Amber's performances take place online. The dolls, doll owners, and viewers—as they post their comments—all become part of the work. When Amber was first posting videos of Amber Doll, people wrote about how much hotter the doll body was than her organic body; they said she was narcissistic for creating a doll in her image. Amber simply let the projections ride. When art flips viewer and viewee like this, we're no longer critiquing the subjects of the art; we're forced to consider the culture that creates and sustains the subjects. It becomes aesthetic empathy in the original sense: we are the Doric column, and the Doric column is us.

The impulse to create art is often the impulse to understand something, to get inside an idea or a character or a hidden part of oneself and make meaning from that understanding. It's an empathic impulse. When Amber first ordered Amber Doll, she had just graduated from art school, where she said she didn't fit in at all. Her peers came from Ivy League schools, whereas she had worked in fashion and been in a sorority. She was "stumbling out as queer" but couldn't find a meaningful relationship. She saw kinship in this outsider community of doll owners who experienced similar failed attempts with women but had found a way to get their needs filled, which she realized was "pretty brilliant." She said she "felt like [Amber Doll] was some or many answers" to her relationship problems and to the dichotomy of victim and victimizer she wanted to explore in her art.

Amber lived with Amber Doll for close to two years. She never had sex with her because in public performances, "everyone understood her body as sexually available with three penetrable orifices so people would explore her violently . . . that interrupted my desire for her body." She definitely loved Amber Doll, though. She moved her and dressed her and cleaned her, and through this connected with the doll husbands.

"They saw that I did care for Amber Doll, that I was interested in generally agreed-upon maintenance," she said, adding that she'd ask the men about various cleaning techniques or the chemical compounds used for repairs. She also says that a flip side of empathy is manipulation; when you listen deeply to someone, you understand their needs. "I think it's vulnerable for people to express needs, and I work hard to not take the manipulation path. I do think that had I gone that route of representing them before they asked me to, it would have felt manipulative to me."

In writing, I've found, it's nearly impossible to fully hate the characters you create—even when their behaviors are loathsome on the page. The very act of writing them necessitates a kind of curiosity, which in itself becomes a kind of love, and the more fully fleshed the characters grow, the less capable they are of unidimensional motive.

This is true of nonfiction as well as fiction; the parent, sibling, or politician you can't stand in real life becomes someone more complicated once you have tried to live in their minds and then reanimate them through literature. When I write about Seth, I'm faithful to my understanding of his temperament and his changes, but I'm also aware that it's just my understanding, and a space opens up for a more real person to enter my very real life.

It's the same, I imagine, with something like a doll; you may at first hate the misogyny she represents—and the misogyny may always be there—but once you make art with her, you care for her wellbeing. Art making, then, becomes a model for the kind of paradox that Baldwin espoused: we can expose violations while caring for the violators, especially when we see that the violator is also inside of us. This, to me, seems like a most radical and propitious empathy.

Amber, however, is adamant that empathy is about not taking a direct or personal stance. She doesn't want to make judgments but rather listen carefully to various conversations and provide venues for those conversations to replicate and transform. It makes me think of Dian and the nonviolent communication class, where direct repetition of speech can shift both the message and the messenger.

The Amber Doll project is now nearly a decade old. I visited Amber-as-Tilikum where she lies on a table next to Lolita in the artist's studio. Amber's considered a burial at sea for both sculptures, but she isn't sure when or how. For now, she's working on commissioning a second Amber Doll with her older face and, for the first time ever, a silicone body scaled to a living human's precise shape. Amber's working with the doll studio to replicate her scars and tattoos, belly fat and cellulite. Her new ideas are less about victims and confinement and more about permission and consent. She plans to give this second self away.

JUST AS AMBER'S WORK gestures toward earlier feminist art but also moves beyond it, I think the current focus on empathy is doing something new. As in the past, a particular discovery—this time it was the mirror neurons—led the trend away from the selfish hypothesis and back toward the belief that we're social creatures. That spurred interest in empathy across multiple fields. There are battles over whether empathy is a skill or an orientation (I prefer the latter), and how best to model it and maximize it for children and others. But what empathy *does* or should do—that's where things get really interesting. In this current iteration of empathy everything, we're seeing a movement toward consciously integrating empathy in the public sphere, rather than confining it to one-on-one interactions between people or a person and an object. Performances are a part of that, and so are classrooms, but increasingly there are calls for empathy in courtrooms and communities, police units and governing bodies. This brings us to questions of how empathy functions differently in different contexts, and whether empathy can be, at root, a force for good.

· PART II ·

Justice

5

Courting Empathy

Six years ago, on Halloween, I was violently attacked while waiting for a train at the Fourteenth Street subway station in New York City. My assailants were multiple, about seven or eight teenagers in a big noisy group, all wearing costumes and masks for the holiday. They called me names and shoved me from behind, bashing my face into a wall. As they ran away and I crumpled to the ground, my first thought was, "Those could be my students."

I'm a college professor, but I've also taught high school, and I've spent most of my professional career researching and writing about urban teenagers. Because of their (sometimes ludicrous) honesty, their hope, and their resilience, they're my favorite demographic. So even as the kids left me to wait for an ambulance in a dirty subway puddle of my blood, I made up stories about who they were. I humanized them almost instantly, made them fit a rubric I understood (*my* students) to ease the confusion of an entirely alien attack.

A day later, the detective assigned to my case pressed me solely for the physical details of my assailants, and while I told him I had only seen their rubber masks and capes, he still made racist assumptions. I was angry at his bigotry and his plan to cultivate a lineup, as I've known several innocent people subjected to this kind of humiliation. And even if he could have found them, I didn't want what the cop wanted: I didn't want those kids to be punished. What I wanted,

I thought back then, was to get them in a room and talk to them. Like a teacher. A teacher with questionable pedagogy perhaps, but a teacher nonetheless.

In my fantasy room alone with my (restrained) assailants, I first wanted to yell at them, and then talk. The kids had called me a dyke as they beat me, so what they committed was a hate crime, and initially I wanted to shout out every hateful epithet I could think of to get even and to make them feel as small and scared as I had that night. I wanted to see if they'd feel sorry if they knew whom they were beating, if they saw a *human being* behind the idea they punished. And then, I wanted to listen, to see if I could understand their motivations. Because if I could understand them, even just a bit, then I would sense our shared humanity and New York wouldn't feel so scary anymore.

I've thought a lot about that Halloween since then. And I've wondered if I'm among an isolated minority who would seek communication rather than retribution. I've thought that maybe my reaction came out of my studies in criminal justice and the way I know that jail time, especially with youth offenders, doesn't repair any root dysfunction and can lead to a terrible pattern of lifelong recidivism. But then my reaction was so immediate and instinctive: I wondered if something deeper was at play.

Even though my assailants would never be found, I started reading about victim-offender mediation programs and discovered that I was far from the minority in seeking out this type of remediation after this type of crime. The programs started proliferating in the late 1970s, and there are now more than 250 across the country, in every state—and they're expanding all the time. At the heart of every program is an empathic exchange, a grasp at understanding: "Who are you, and why did you do this to me?"

In this way, empathy makes its way out of the one-to-one exchanges of babies and children or interpersonal nonviolent communication and into public life. Even as the courtroom players may be individual, they've entered the realm of public spectacle and precedent, and empathy plays the hinge in the move toward justice. But the questions many are asking are these: Is a courtroom precisely *not* the place for empathy? Does empathy create bias? Should justice be blind? Or is our criminal justice system exactly where we need empathy the most?

While mediation (sometimes called restitution or restorative justice) programs are nearing their fifty-year anniversary, their roots are much older. Our current American system comes from the British one, which, until King Henry I, had been restitutional in nature. In medieval England, crimes and their prosecution were handled locally by voluntary organizations called tithings. When someone was robbed, for instance, the victim would notify their tithing, which would pursue the thief and make him give the money back. If the thief couldn't or wouldn't, the tithing would allow the victim to seek revenge. The point is, the victim was the focal point: the whole purpose of justice was to make the victim whole again.

King Henry I, black-haired and barrel-chested, was the youngest son of William the Conqueror (or William the Bastard, if you asked a Brit), who had seized England for the Normans. When William died, Henry promptly crowned himself king and set about changing everything in the consolidated lands.

Mainly, Henry needed money to protect his kingdom. His father had initiated a system of taxes on landowners, and Henry bureaucratized it, appointing royal justices to tour the shires and demand payment, usually aggressively. These appointees were often lowborn men who suddenly had power and rank, and the right to visit or inspect the holdings of virtually anyone with land.

It was at this moment that the notion of justice, restitution, and retribution shifted dramatically.

King Henry's tax collectors were enforcing law from the *outside* — visiting shires and towns and demanding payment for the crown. Soon, as law men, they were adjudicating criminal disputes as well—previously handled by the tithings—as they realized the justice process was a new fount of funds. They determined crimes were against the "king's peace" rather than against an individual victim, and thus all fines and penalties could be directed to the kingdom. The tithings, and the victim's legal centrality, disappeared.

In many ways, Henry's model has stuck. We've replaced the king with the state, and a crime is defined as an offense against a public law. The victim, if anything, is a side note: proof only that a crime occurred. Over time, restitution gave way to retribution as criminals couldn't pay and we began to lock people in prisons for crimes against the state. Over time, the dialogue between victim and criminal was lost completely.

Restorative justice is still practiced in some pockets of the world, and as it's quietly reemerging as an option in first-world cities with overcrowded prisons filled with recidivist inmates, teenagers seem to be the programs' primary guinea pigs. There are more victim-offender mediation programs in juvenile courts than in their adult counterparts, perhaps because people imagine kids are easier to restore.

"Across multiple courts, there's more openness to being more empathic to young people and to seeing them as part of their environments, and to send them to untraditional programs," says Kate Barrow, director of the Alternatives to Incarceration Program at the Red Hook Community Justice Center in Brooklyn. Barrow runs untraditional programming at a very untraditional courthouse. Red Hook is the first multijurisdictional court in the nation, meaning it houses criminal, housing, and family court under one roof, with one judge presiding. Traditionally, people cycle through some or all of these courts without any of their cases overlapping, and without any one person understanding the root causes. For instance, a drug addiction may lead a person to theft and criminal court. If she does jail time or incurs a fee, she might fall behind in her rent and land in housing court. If she goes to a homeless shelter and the children miss school, she'll be in family court. These three separate sentences take her time and attention away from dealing with her core problem. If her jurisdiction is in Red Hook, though, the judge will know her more integrated story. And he can sentence her with the catch-all penalty of mandated rehab. Twelve years into Red Hook's opening, the center launched the Adolescent Diversion Program. If this woman's kids are acting out from all the dislocation and trauma

say, they start stealing or fighting in school—they can be offered counseling, tutoring, community service, or a version of restorative justice Red Hook calls the Peacemaking Program.

In the courtroom itself, there's a district attorney who, as in any other court, represents the government in prosecuting criminal offenses. Barrow says the DA is more likely to agree to this kind of diversionary sentencing with adolescents than adults—and ultimately wipe the case off a kid's record.

"There's a greater ability to put oneself in a teenager's shoes. People can say, 'I can remember being volatile and disrespectful when I was a teenager,'" Barrow said from her office at the courthouse. It felt cozy there with high windows, a blue-and-white rug, and a tapestry on the wall. "Whereas we often perceive an adult as a hardened criminal. We think of someone who is making rational decisions about his life. There's a different desire for accountability."

I watched several cases unfold one afternoon at the Red Hook court. The building used to be a Catholic school, and the white walls, blonde wood floors, and enormous windows everywhere give the place an exalted, airy feel; it's nothing like the overly fluorescent, scuffed courts downtown. The interior of the school had been completely gutted; the holding cells have glass walls instead of bars, and unlike any other court I've ever seen, the judge wasn't on an elevated platform of any kind. He wore his robes, but his bench was a simple desk, at eye level with everybody else.

The day I visited, Judge Alex Calabrese was hearing criminal cases, both juvenile and adult. The courtroom deputy, a large white bald man with a bushy moustache in the shape of a frown, would bellow out a name and number and somebody would shuffle forward with one of the Legal Aid lawyers who stood to the side of the room. At the other side were a couple of district attorneys, and in the middle of it all was Alvin, a black man with a hearty laugh in a maroon turtleneck and black suit. Alvin is the resource coordinator: every day, before clients appear in court, they go upstairs to meet with the alternative sanctions and clinical folks who assess their needs— be it GED, mental health, employment, whatever—and determine their compliance with past court mandates. Over the heads of the lawyers, Alvin communicates all this with the judge.

"We recommended nine peacemaking sessions to you," Judge Calabrese said to a skinny boy with a polka dot backpack who had approached the bar. Alvin, glancing through a folder, nodded his assent. "And sixteen counseling sessions. Did you do it?"

Through his lawyer, the boy (I'll call him Michael) asserted that he had. Although we were technically in criminal court, Calabrese knew many of the families who passed through because of housing or family matters or just from being in the neighborhood. In this case, Michael's grandmother had died, after which fights with his mother escalated. Once, things got physical. His mother called the police, and Michael was arrested. Michael chose to do peacemaking rather than a stint in juvenile hall, and two or three neutral peacemakers met with him and his mother over the many sessions to let them each talk. The peacemaking system is based on a Navajo model (each restorative justice program is slightly different) with a talking stick and storytelling and no judgments. The idea is that both defendant and the complainant witness speak as long as they're holding the stick, with no interruption, often excavating history that dates back long before the inciting incident. The peacemaking coordinator at Red Hook told me she's referred about 140 cases a year, but only about 40 actually follow through. Of these, 90 percent are crimes committed within families. Store owners who have been burglarized, for instance, have shown interest in peacemaking but usually ultimately back out.

After the peacemakers have aired their grievances and backstories, they discuss "healing steps" to restitute the crime, the relationship, the community, whatever's been harmed. After Alvin whispered in Calabrese's ear, the judge said to Michael, "I hear you've been doing tours of colleges." This was one of Michael's healing steps. "Have you decided where you might want to go?"

Michael grinned. He gave the judge a list of schools, and Calabrese asked him to approach the bench. "On behalf of the DA, Peacemaking, your lawyers and your mother, this case is dismissed and sealed," Calabrese said. The assault would never appear on his record. He handed Michael a blue folder. "You've been working very hard, and I'd like to give you a certificate of accomplishment."

The courtroom broke into applause, and Michael tucked himself beneath Calabrese's outstretched arm for a photo. I tried to imagine my subway assailants adopting such a pose but couldn't; I hadn't even seen their faces. I didn't know if any of the kids would have wanted to make friends with a judge and peace with their conscience. Was the attack led by one bully? Was it a dare, a plot, or a spontaneous burst of teenage rage suddenly tunneling in on one target they could topple? That night, at the hospital, there were sixteen other victims of gay bashing; the rumor was that gangs used the Halloween parade as an initiation site.

I would never know my attackers' motivations or their backstories, but I continued to meet with, and write about, other troubled, angry teenagers as a way, in part, to imbue the violence with meaning. I couldn't accept that I had been randomly objectified, as that erasure cut more deeply than being seen and singled out. Victim-offender reconciliation programs in Canada and the United States are very often property cases, with burglary being a main offense. In the eyes of the law, these are small crimes, suitable for potential remediation. But in the eyes of the victim, burglary is felt personally.

If your house has been robbed, you may have felt as I did. You want to know who did it, and why, and whether they plan to strike somebody else down the line.

THE FIRST DOCUMENTED CASE of restorative justice in North America was in Ontario in 1974. After two young men vandalized twenty-two properties, their probation officers marched them around to the property owners to seek amends. The probation officers were Mennonite, and other Mennonite thinkers took up the practice, including author Howard Zehr, now considered the grandfather of restorative justice. The movement incorporated other theologies and perspectives, including aboriginal and Native American traditions, and now restorative justice is often taught as a component of criminal justice programs all across the continent. In New Zealand, all juvenile cases are handled with a restorative model, and more locally, smaller jurisdictions have voted to adopt the cause. In Colorado, the governor approved a pilot program in four counties for juvenile cases, whereby all victims, offenders, law enforcement officials, and community members will meet in a "circle process" to speak about their experiences, understand the harm, and decide on the actions for restitution.

Most of the other restorative justice programs, like Peacemaking at the Red Hook court, are voluntary in nature. But they all, at base, ask a very different set of questions than traditional criminal justice. That approach demands to know what law was broken, who did it, and what punishment he deserves. Restorative justice involves a lot more people and looks to understand cause. Restorative justice, according to Zehr, asks,

1. Who has been hurt?
2. What are their needs?
3. Whose obligations are these?
4. What are the causes?

5. Who has a stake in the situation?
6. What is the appropriate process to involve stakeholders in an effort to address causes and put things right?

RESTORATIVE JUSTICE, in other words, tries to weave a web of understanding and repair. It's messier than the decontextualized, one-two punch of crime and consequence. It's a humanized, empathic approach to what is, by design, the passionless metrics of the law. Some say that approach is very dangerous.

In most violent crimes like mine, victims know nothing about their offenders. Details about their childhoods, early suffering or abuse, addictions, or even past crimes are inadmissible in court. Only the victim's lawyer gets to cross-examine the defendant, and then, only about specifics pertaining to the incident at hand. Any context or motivation for the crime is considered, at best, irrelevant and, at worst, as inducing bias. Traditionally, the only time the victim is allowed to speak on her own terms is once the verdict has been reached, in a prepared "victim impact statement" during or after sentencing, and the offender doesn't get to respond at all.

My daughter's childhood best friend was the offender in a violent crime; she's now serving twenty-five years in a maximum security prison in California. Angela's case followed standard protocol: she was issued a Legal Aid lawyer, she wasn't offered any restorative justice, and she's now paying off mandated fees to the victim's family in the form of a prison job where she earns bit change by the hour. According to the court records, Angela and a boyfriend stole a car and drove to a 7-Eleven, where they held up a lone employee at gunpoint. For four hours, they held this man hostage while they drank beers from the fridge until the cops finally raided the store and arrested them both.

While the employee was physically unhurt, I imagine he was terrified. Perhaps he had nightmares, perhaps the holdup impacted his ability to work or earn money. He didn't issue a victim statement so I can't know. But I do know some of Angela's story, both before and after the crime, and I wonder if he could have understood a bit more about her life—if he could have felt some empathy—his terrible night might have left a less permanent scar. This is a fantasy, of course, based on my wish to empathize with my own attackers, to resonate with some strand of their lives so I could live in the world of humans like me and not monsters.

Angela now feels bad about what she did, though on the night of the crime she was flying high on crack. She had been using for a few years, as a way to both escape the pain of her childhood and to understand her birthmother. Back when she was just smoking pot, Angela had said to me that she couldn't comprehend the way a mother would choose drugs over her own children. Angela's early home life had been a series of motel rooms as her mother chased her highs; as a six-year-old, she was begging for food at bodegas. When the state caught up with them, and Angela and her younger brother were placed in foster care, her life didn't improve by much. She was still shuffled through different homes and different families with people who didn't want her. Finally, she and her brother ended up with someone who said he'd be a permanent parent until Angela hit her teens, and then he only wanted her brother.

Like my daughter, Angela is transgender, and her foster father was overwhelmed by her transition. When I met Angela, she was living with a foster mom who accepted her, but by then Angela was testing any adult who claimed to care for her, she had been burned so many times. She was skipping school and doing drugs, and she stole a car for a joyride, just to see how it would feel to be chased by the cops. Angela's foster mother dutifully attended her mounting juvenile court hearings, but she made her one promise: if Angela were arrested as an adult, her loyalty would end.

Just after her eighteenth birthday, Angela tested this promise at the 7-Eleven. At her trial, they called her a "man who impersonates a woman." To the end, nobody saw Angela for what she was.

If the judge had known Angela's story like I had, would he have handed down a twenty-five-year sentence? Would he have known she'd already been taking hormones for years, and that remanding her to a men's prison was condemning her to a self-imposed solitary confinement? Or would he have mustered empathy and doled out a safer landing?

IN 2009, PRESIDENT BARACK OBAMA needed to replace a Supreme Court justice, and he listed empathy as a primary criterion. Political pandemonium ensued. Empathy, the senators, analysts, and academics cried, has no place in the courtroom. The law is rational and applied equally to all, and empathy can skew law's inherent impartiality. When Obama nominated Sonia Sotomayor, her old speeches and judgments were scrutinized in a hunt for signs of potential empathy. It was a word that had come to mean, strangely, leaning toward one side or the other. As Maryland senator Ben Cardin said in an interview, "In terms of ruling from the bench, there really isn't a role for empathy to play."

In a widely quoted lecture delivered to students eight years prior, Sotomayor had said, "I would hope that a wise Latina woman with the richness of her experiences would more often than not reach a better conclusion than a white male who hasn't lived that life." Some called Sotomayor a racist, while others argued that Sotomayor was speaking a simple and obvious truth — that nobody, judge or otherwise, can expect to wrench himself from his background. Neutrality was an ideal, but it was a myth.

Ultimately, in her four days of Senate hearings, Sotomayor was repeatedly grilled about whether she would let feelings or experiences influence her decisions. Although she herself had never even used the word "empathy," she said, "I wouldn't approach the issue of judging the way the president does . . . It's not the heart that compels conclusions in cases, it's the law." The committee's ranking Republican said that "it was good to see the nominee renounce the Obama empathy test."

Today, the test still stands. All District/Circuit Court nominees are asked about the role that empathy plays in their worldview and in their court decisions.

Judge Calabrese doesn't think of his work at Red Hook in terms of empathy. Even though his court offers services in lieu of jail time, he says he thinks more about the interplay of a defendant's needs versus community safety.

"If I see someone who is in possession of drugs and every other case seems to be a robbery of the first degree where they're supporting their drug habit by pointing guns in people's faces, I'm not going to give them the chance to do treatment," Calabrese said. He had finished with his cases for the afternoon and come to find me in the tiny Peacemaking office, where two desks filled a room the size of a closet. He had taken off his robes, and his grey suit matched his carefully combed hair. He's short, broad-shouldered, and plainspoken — the kind of guy who won't take punches but whose eyes crinkle merrily when he laughs.

"I understand that there may be lots of reasons fueling their use of drugs. It may be, as a kid, they experienced some traumatic things and they've been addicted since age thirteen or twelve," he said. "But it's not a question of not being empathetic to them or not understanding the situation. It's a question of safety. Because some people need to be incarcerated is the only way to put it."

Earlier in the day, I watched a case that, to me, seemed to teeter right along safety's edge. It was an assault case, and the defendant was a teenager dressed in tight jeans and a big red sweatshirt. She looked furious. Every time her lawyer whispered something in her ear, she scowled and kicked at the floor. I'll call her Sephina. Apparently, earlier that year, Sephina had beat up a classmate. Then she attacked a teacher. Both times, she'd been sent to Calabrese, and he remanded her to mental health treatment. Now, though, she'd assaulted the principal. The school was demanding a full order of protection and the DA wanted to set a three-thousand-dollar bail.

Sephina's lawyer, a harried-looking woman with a short pony-tail, said that her client was willing to undergo more intensive therapy at her clinic. Calabrese thumbed through a file on his desk and then looked up. "Here's what I don't understand," he said, pointing to the file. "She was scheduled for therapy and she missed it. She was scheduled again and she missed it. How can she go for more inten-sive treatment if she's not going for treatment-treatment?"

The lawyer asked to approach the bench and whispered some-thing to Calabrese. Alvin, the resource coordinator, loped up to me and whispered too. "Here's a kid who's beat up three people, and now he's going to give her even more treatment," he said. He knew what the judge was planning to do; he'd seen it all before. "That's some empathy."

Now Calabrese addressed Sephina directly. His voice was low and stern. "The DA has asked me to require three-thousand-dol-lar bail on this case. Do you understand what this means?" Sephina didn't answer; she just squared her shoulders and stared hard into the middle distance. Calabrese continued. "It means this is serious. It means you would have sat in jail until someone paid your bail. But this is not going to go on your record or affect your future. We're giving you an opportunity to treat it. We're going to work with you to contact Community Counseling and Mediation tomorrow—"

"Today, Your Honor," Alvin interrupted. "We're going to call them today!"

Sephina continued to stand, rooted and rigid and mad, and I re-alized she was a perfect argument for excising empathy from court-rooms. After all, in mock trials, juries recommend lighter sentences only for defendants who express sadness. A philosopher named Jesse

Prinz has argued against summoning empathy in moral decision-making because empathetic accuracy—our ability to correctly identify someone else's emotions—increases when that person is viewed as attractive. Prinz writes about "cuteness effects" (we're more likely to feel empathy for a mouse than a rat, say) and suggests these effects could be extended to human beings. Since the teenager on trial was neither sad nor particularly cute, I thought it was important that the judge not dock her for her attitude. Perhaps Sephina's emotional armor was hard-earned and vital to her survival; she was so different from Angela, with Angela's softness and tears and longing for love, but both girls deserved the same shot at rehabilitation.

I was grateful for the notion of blind justice as the judge and Alvin discussed schools that might accept this girl with a violent past, in time for her to take the Regents exam. I could argue that Calabrese was adopting an entirely neutral, unempathetic approach to this case: if he could push for services for this hard, untouchable teenager, he would push for everyone equally. But then there's another idea. Some theorists argue that judges ought to *develop* their capacity for empathy in order to become more impartial, more fair and evenhanded.

In the *University of Cincinnati Law Review,* law professor Rebecca K. Lee writes that judges historically are an elite group and may unconsciously favor the advantaged party in a dispute. White judges, she points out, are more likely to let a part of a plaintiff's employment discrimination case move past summary judgment if the plaintiff is white than if he is not. It takes a conscious empathy, she argues, to uncover this kind of internalized bias. Judges need to make a concentrated effort to understand others' experiences from their perspectives—especially when they're dramatically different than their own—in order to make the court a level playing field.

Lee cites Martha C. Nussbaum, the feminist philosopher who writes extensively on law and ethics, who says judges should be "judicious spectators." As such, Nussbaum writes, they need to go "beyond empathy," measuring the suffering of anyone implicated in a case. I don't know how much Nussbaum Judge Calabrese has read, but at one point during the teenager's trial, he asked if family court was involved. Sephina's lawyer said her mother and aunt had been in court all day. I had noticed the women earlier and figured they were related; they were sitting behind me but when the assault case was called, I could hear one of them crying.

I went back to sit with them. "I have a daughter too," I whispered. I remembered when Angela had stolen the car and my daughter Christina was in the front seat beside her. Christina's record was cleared, but I too had sat in a courthouse for hours, scared and lonely, unsure what a guilty verdict would mean for both of our futures.

And maybe this is what Nussbaum means when she writes about measuring the suffering of everyone implicated; maybe it was why Calabrese asked if there was family in the room before he recommended therapy over bail.

Later, in the hallway, this mother told me how grateful she was for Red Hook Community Court. "It's so much better than criminal court where they just send you off to Rikers, which is so bad for a sixteen- or seventeen-year-old. Here they help you," she said. Just then, her daughter emerged from the courtroom, led by Alvin. Her mother reached for her, but Sephina marched straight past her, her eyes steely and set straight ahead. "We've been here all day," the mom said sadly, letting herself collapse against the wall. "Everybody needs help."

Alvin and Sephina would pass the youth and community programs room with its giant mural created by kids who had been caught doing graffiti. They would head upstairs past an intake desk with a sign reading, "I'm here to help you," and down a hall lined with art, passing the GED classroom, private counseling rooms, and finally into the bright and airy room of caseworkers, whose cubicles were filled with plants, peace posters, and framed photos of their kids. Here, Sephina would draw up her latest, and hopefully final, plan for treatment.

"What I love about Red Hook is that the same people who, if you went down to 120 Schermerhorn Street [a traditional criminal court], you'd see getting thirty-day jail, we can work with and be successful," Calabrese said to me. In an independent study, auditors showed that a defendant whose case was processed at Red Hook faced a 20 percent lower risk of rearrest than a defendant whose case was processed in a traditional court. A youth faced a 30 percent lower risk. Crime in the Red Hook catchment area also decreased significantly after the court opened in 2000 and has stayed low. Part of this is due to the fact that housing, family, and criminal court are all housed together, and Calabrese can look at a defendant's complete records to better understand, and treat, his needs. To oversee jurisdiction in all three courts, Calabrese had to be named an acting Supreme Court justice — something other judges could do, but so far, none has tried. Said Calabrese, "What to you is reason, logic, and common sense is to the court system, rocket science."

The other reason behind Red Hook's success is the nature of a community court itself. The first was launched as an experiment in midtown Manhattan in 1993. There are now thirty-seven community courts around the United States and thirty-three in other countries. Each one is slightly different, but the basic premise is that rather than just being a site that sentences offenders, the court should operate as a part of the community and as an agent of transformation within it. For instance, at Red Hook, the court is involved in a community farm and a local theater. It sponsors movie nights and a youth baseball league, and provides internships and arts classes. At all community courts, there's more of a focus on learning about each defendant, creating individualized justice, and providing a wider range of options outside of jail time and fines. (The majority of defendants do restitution in the form of community service or receive social services or drug treatment.) The court's success is measured by overall crime reduction within the community.

Most of the arguments against harnessing empathy in criminal justice aren't posited in this context of community. They focus on the ways a singular defendant in a singular courtroom might be favored over another kind of defendant. Paul Bloom, for instance, is a psychology and cognitive science professor at Yale who's written several articles and now a book arguing against empathy as a moral policy guide. Bloom calls empathy "parochial, narrow-minded, and innumerate" and argues for the "reasoned, even counter-empathetic analysis of moral obligation." Utilizing reason over the "gut wrench of empathy" will keep us from over-identifying with traumatized victims or baby-faced offenders. In the bigger picture, it will help us make sound policies affecting the many over the few. Empathy also has a proximity effect; we're more likely to care about the tornado victims one town over than tsunami victims several countries away. Making judicial policies based on reason ensures we strive to value human lives equally, unswayed by our all too human hearts.

But reason isn't an abstraction, a mathematical construct, an immutable natural law. Reason, like empathy, is human and varied, deeply contingent on the person employing it. One's reason is built in moments, culled from school, from family, from weighing ideas and experiences against one another. Your reasoning is not mine, simply because our lives are different, and to employ reason as a sole criterion for justice is to imply that thoughts are extractable from their thinkers.

I could argue that the pro- and anti-empathy philosophers are both fighting for the same end in criminal justice: they want the judges to see beyond their immediate allegiances and biases to ensure a broader kind of fairness. One side says they need to apply empathy to their blind spots; the other says they need to apply a logical, rational outlook. Both, I think, can work, probably in tandem.

At the Red Hook courthouse, one of the last cases Judge Calabrese saw was a woman with over a hundred prior arrests. She was in her early seventies, had no teeth, and evident trouble walking up to the bar. Her last court date was a month earlier, when she tested negative for drugs in her system. This time, Alvin said, she showed trace evidence of cocaine.

Calabrese asked her why she hadn't gone to her treatment program; the woman said her knee had been giving her trouble. But she made it to court for her drug test? Yes, the woman answered shyly, and could she come back again next month? Next time, she promised, she'd be clean.

"You think that some of the value you try to impart actually sticks somewhere in the brain," Calabrese said, adding that the woman simply liked coming in to court to be checked on. She was lonely, and they'd keep working with her to stay in rehab. He said that some of the teenagers who had committed crimes and rejected the court's services later came back to Red Hook of their own accord to get their GEDs. "You continue to work with people and it sticks somewhere along the line."

A Wesleyan philosophy professor and animal ethicist named Lori Gruen writes about empathy in terms of entanglement. She's thinking about human relationships to animals, but it applies, I think, to criminal justice too. Entangled empathy, she says, requires that we already see ourselves as deeply connected to one another. Rather than having empathy for someone we don't immediately understand, or eschewing empathy in favor of a rational, evenhanded morality, Gruen argues, entangled empathy uses both cognition and emotion to recognize our relationships to others, and as such, care about their wellbeing as well as their extended relationships. Entangled empathy, in other words, doesn't just see a defendant and a victim but people with histories who live in families, who live in a neighborhood and a city and a state and a country. They have a relationship with that judge and that jury, who are also in relationship to city and state, and so on. Entangled empathy means considering the fabric as well as the thread.

While he doesn't call it this, I would say that Calabrese is practicing entangled empathy. Ideally, I think our courts would shift toward a more holistic model of justice, wherein we look at whole people rather than singular crimes, and integrate our court much the way Calabrese has done. It's a project that would take tremendous vision and commitment, but at a time when the police, the whip-tail of our justice system, are finally being called out for their entrenched and learned brutality, this is the moment for overhaul.

6

Empathy Traffic

According to Martin Hoffman's developmental stages of empathy, it's around late childhood or early adolescence that we can begin to categorize people into oppressed groups. According to C. Daniel Batson, a social psychologist who spent thirty-some years studying empathy's relationship to altruism, it's easier for people to empathize with, and extend help to, these oppressed or stigmatized groups when we perceive them as victims. But understanding someone's personal responsibility for his stigmatization can undercut the empathy.

Put these ideas together and there's a lot of room for empathy to infantilize, patronize, or reinforce restrictive cultural norms — especially with people wearing shoes we could truly never exchange. Several people have written about the potential colonizing nature of empathy, as the empathizer usually holds the dominant position and can appropriate the other's experience as a means of achieving some personal relief or objective. I thought a lot about these pitfalls while I was in the Red Hook court where the judge, no matter how well-intentioned, definitely had dominance. And to grasp whether groups with unequal power could ever reach an empathic understanding, I realized I had to ask different kinds of questions.

While I was visiting Red Hook Community Justice Center, with its focus on individual offenders in a kind of restorative justice model, an entirely new and unprecedented court was materializing in New York State that focuses on a class of people as a whole. It's called the Human Trafficking Intervention Court (HTIC) and it's for people arrested for prostitution—the first of its kind in the country. And yet it's modeled on other courts and a kind of cultural wave we've been riding for the past twenty-five years. While the United States locks up more people per capita than any other nation on earth, and we are known for our militaristic and brutal police forces, we've also been quietly but steadily trying a different approach with certain sectors of the population. These are the sectors most easily identified as victims, rather than perpetrators, of their crimes. And so, as Batson's research predicts, these are the people who are offered help. As long as they remain victims.

The first of these so-called specialized courts or problem-solving courts was a drug court in Florida; now there are more than 3,400 nationwide. Most of the cases before drug court judges are DWIs or other "victimless" crimes; the victim is the offender himself, who has fallen prey to his addiction and is provided substance abuse treatment. If the offender has been violent or committed a serious felony in thrall to his substance (80 percent of those in jail or prison abuse alcohol or drugs; 50 percent are clinically dependent), he's a criminal and not eligible for drug court.

After drug courts came juvenile drug courts, veterans' courts (which typically provide substance use and anger management programming), and a whole new type of adjudication: domestic violence courts. These last put special emphasis on the victims of intimate partner violence, ensuring their access to community resources and protection.

The timing of this paradigm shift from punishment to helping in circumscribed areas of criminal justice parallels the upswell of all things empathy. And while decreasing jail sentences is undoubtedly useful, this brand of empathy has a note of paternalism. Especially in the latest, and highly contested, prostitution courts.

Like the other specialized courts, the HTICs were launched after judges and other officials noticed the same people getting rearrested, and they realized something in the system was broken. In this case, a judge named Fernando Camacho in Queens saw repeat teenagers he suspected were not doing sex work willingly. They were young; some had pimps; some worked out of brothels; some were citizens, and some were not. Instead of sentencing them, he started referring them to outside agencies that helped victims of sexual violence and trafficking, and in September 2013 the new courts—now utilized for every prostitution arrest in New York State—were born. As Camacho told the Center for Court Innovation, an organization that develops alternative programming for courts across New York State, "The goal is to give prostitutes an opportunity to get out of the life."

The difference with sex workers is some of them may not want to get out. And this is where empathy can falter. The question becomes this: can empathy for an oppressed group actually turn on its head and become another kind of oppression?

"The anti-trafficking movement feels polarized: there's the abolitionist side and the sex workers' rights/empowerment side," said Miriam Goodman, the coordinator for trafficking programs at the Center for Court Innovation. She is also the assistant director of a specific anti-trafficking court in midtown Manhattan. Goodman knows all the facts: more than 100,000 children are trafficked in the United States every year, they're mostly U.S. citizens, and they're lured into the work by pimps or acquaintances who promise them easy money. And then they can't get out.

I knew a teenager who fit this prototype. She was a foster kid, whom I'll call Sarah, without any deep emotional ties to her foster or biological family. Research shows that pimps seek out this kind of child for their brothels and massage parlors, the kids whose families won't come looking for them. Sarah ran away, as foster kids do, and met a cool-looking older girl who told her she knew of a job where the money was fast. The older girl took Sarah to an apartment in Brooklyn where Sarah was locked up and forced to have sex with whatever men came through. Sarah never kept the money she earned. Her pimp was from a local gang, another common occurrence, as gangs are increasingly taking control of sex trafficking. Sarah said she was forced to take drugs to sleep and wake and was beaten when she didn't comply. Her only means of escape was to attempt suicide; the pimp found her too "crazy" for work.

This population of the sex trade, the enslaved and trafficked children, is undoubtedly victimized. It's the population that Judge Camacho identified when the same sixteen-year-old, a girl named Siobhan, appeared before his bench repeatedly and he first decided to provide resources and help. The sticking point, for sex work advocates, is that not all prostitutes are trafficked. These sex workers are still arrested, still often treated badly by the police, still made to go before a judge—all before they're offered a unilateral array of services, services some of them don't want. This is the problem when empathy veers into altruism or helping, as it so often does: helping becomes about the helper's goals. Trafficking court began with an empathic attention to some people's needs, leading to a broad-based attempt to fulfill those needs, which may have led in turn to a blurring out of the original population.

At least this was my question as I met with Miriam Goodman and sat in the new court talking with sex workers and trauma therapists. Does a system designed to only help victims help people who don't see themselves as victims at all?

"Our expectations have changed. The help we assumed they wanted isn't always the help they want," Goodman said. I met her at the Midtown Community Court, where prostitution cases are held on Tuesdays. The court itself is on the first floor of a six-story building; client services are on the fourth floor, and therapy groups are held in the basement. The building is encased in scaffolding (according to Goodman it's been under construction "forever"), and it also houses a theater; bits of old wooden sets lean against available walls. On the docket the day I visited were thirty prostitution arrests, mixed in among other "quality of life" crimes like panhandling or jumping subway turnstiles. All told, the judge would see about fifty cases, which was typical. Most of the new arrests for sex work would get the same mandate: six counseling sessions, both private and in group.

It's in these counseling sessions, Goodman said, that she and other therapists can break from the one-size-fits-all model of a judge's mandate and hopefully provide real assistance. "I've personally worked with the most pimp-controlled women chained to a pole in the basement and then I've worked with Columbia grad students who are paying off their debt. Neither of these people might identify as a victim of trafficking, but they might need certain things," Goodman observed. She is short and slight, with straight brown hair and big, grey glasses; she has a bookish, serious demeanor, though she also laughs abruptly and easily. This is a happy surprise, like a bowlful of apples in a law library.

Goodman realizes it's important that her team is transparent with all the clients that come through. Thus, they utilize the federal definition of trafficking. The Trafficking Victims Protection Act defines "severe acts of trafficking in persons" as "the recruitment, harboring, transportation, provision, or obtaining of a person for the purpose of a commercial sex act, in which the commercial sex act is induced by force, fraud, or coercion, or in which the person induced to perform such act has not attained 18 years of age." This, Goodman knows, does not fit all sex workers, not by any stretch. But still, she said, "once people learn about trafficking, sometimes they do identify with it."

Whether they do or they don't, however, is less important to Goodman than meeting people where they're at. She says her clients have the right to define themselves. And even if they do meet the criteria for trafficking, she understands that they may not be able to meet the mandate for counseling. "She may never want to because of drugs or because her pimp is her intimate partner," Goodman said. "But she may want her GED and you can help her with that." Helping someone, in other words, doesn't necessarily follow from empathizing with them or being able to imagine yourself in those shoes and where those shoes *should* be walking.

MIDTOWN COMMUNITY COURT has none of the airy open feeling of the Red Hook courtroom; it's crowded and fluorescent, with brown floor tiles and scuffed wooden seats, banked on both sides with old filing cabinets. A substitute judge named Lisa Sokoloff presided at a raised bench, and most cases took under two minutes to conclude. Most everything's in code: prostitution cases are "AP-8s," arrests are "undercover shield 285," and defendants are offered "ACDs." Woman after woman (and that day, all the sex workers were women) walked to the bar, as Sokoloff described their cases as a series of letters and numbers and then dismissed them to their mandated counseling. It was about as exciting as a day at the DMV.

Goodman sat next to me and translated. An "undercover shield 285" was a plainclothes cop, and an ACD stood for "adjournment in contemplation of dismissal," which meant that if the defendant completed her mandate and wasn't rearrested, her case would be dismissed in six months. Every neighborhood is different, but midtown has a lot of hotels and massage parlors, so most of the sex work happens indoors, and the arrests are made by undercover officers. Many of the women arrested in midtown are Chinese, and the court offers translators for Mandarin, Spanish, Korean, and Wolof.

As soon as Judge Sokoloff dismissed an AP-8 defendant, a senior counselor and anti-trafficking coordinator at the court, Jamie Bedard, would step up to meet her and escort her to the fourth floor to set up her counseling. Bedard is tall and blonde with an open, friendly face. I met her in the basement room where she holds group therapy sessions; it was a freezing, cinder-block space with exposed pipes and old boxes crammed in the corner. An armed guard stood outside the door.

"It's a real positive that we can sit in this cold, dingy, terrible dungeon room with a court officer outside so people feel they're being perp walked—and then provide an environment of acceptance," Bedard said. Most of the time, she explained, she starts her group sessions by breaking down stereotypes; participants list words like "prostitute" or "pimp," "social worker" and "john," as well as what society tends to think about those words. Then they talk about possible realities for people who are labeled that way. This is a safe way, Jamie argues, for people to share their stories without necessarily claiming them as their own. "They feel less alone, which to me is such a huge marker of success."

Goodman, who was in the dungeon therapy room with us, chimed in. "I think it's that they're often put in situations where it's unsafe to trust other girls, whether it's in foster care group homes or with pimps." Most of the individual therapy is conducted by women, and the groups are almost always all female-identified. At first the counselors thought about moving the therapy offsite, away from the dungeon and the guard, but the women said they wanted to have their sessions at the courthouse; it was a place their pimps or boyfriends couldn't get to them. Goodman and Bedard were also surprised, at first, by how little the clients claimed they had ever shared about themselves before being mandated to do it. Goodman said, "Mostly they just haven't been asked questions in a safe, supported way. It's really wonderful that they have this space but it's also really sad that it took this"—she gestured up toward the courtroom—"to start talking."

After examining stereotypes, the women in group therapy discuss safety within the life of prostitution, healthy boundaries and relationships, and they learn about trauma and affect regulation. Pro bono financial planners and criminal and immigration attorneys run sessions on financial literacy and legal rights. But before all this,

Bedard or an intern holds a one-on-one counseling session—immediately after the woman's hearing.

"It's so jarring for people to go from the court environment, where you're not too sure what happened and the attorney didn't have an hour to sit with you, and then to come upstairs and feel safe and accepted," Bedard said, explaining that sometimes she sets up a future date for a client, but very often, they want to talk right there. "I try to get a sense of what brought them here, where they're living, but people spend a good bit of time talking about their upbringing. I think they're caught off guard and they share."

I talked with one sex worker, a young woman who was willing to be interviewed but wanted to be called "B-Blah" for the record. B —I'll call her B—had gone upstairs to see Bedard but had scheduled her private session for another day; she just wanted to get a sandwich and go back to her friend's house. B had already been arrested and had been through the group sessions before; she said the counseling could be "good for some people but others won't take it to heart or take it in and they'll just do it all over again; it depends on the person."

B was twenty-six and from Indiana. She appreciated that the courts here "didn't want to see people locked up" and were more "lenient" than what she'd seen back home. Still, she expected to be arrested again, as legal work wasn't on her radar. "I need to get a whole lot of things before I could do that," she said. "A place to live, a name change. A husband."

B reminded me of a lot of girls I've known; she was polite to the judge but irreverent and sassy on the street. She smiled at me when she turned around in court, which was part of the reason I felt comfortable approaching her later. The other reason was that the judge had called out B's male name. I've been in countless bureaucratic situations with my daughter, my partner, or friends when they've been misnamed or misgendered, and I know how soul-stripping it can be. I felt for her.

B, however, thought the experience was fine: "In New York City, there are a lot of people who are transgender. I don't think it's as harsh here as other courts might be because they know what's going on." Her trajectory was familiar to me. Like a lot of young transgender people, she left a small town for a big city on the coast in the hopes of finding a community. Once she got there, she couldn't work without some form of legal female ID—something that's now possible to procure, but it takes time and resources. In the meantime, she had to eat. Transpeople of color like B face tremendous employment discrimination: they have an unemployment rate four times the national average. (Transpeople in general are four times as likely to have an income under ten thousand dollars per year, and 90 percent have experienced harassment or discrimination on the job.) B fell into sex work as the fastest and most available option.

B is not a victim of trafficking; she doesn't have a pimp and works for herself. The courts connect clients with the city's limited housing and shelter resources, and Bedard said they often refer clients like B to an LGBT program, which could probably offer her help with a name-change. Still, when I told her about a nonprofit dedicated to IDs, she hadn't heard of it. Besides, what she needed was more than any of the court's resources could provide: she needed to live in a different kind of society overall.

ALTHOUGH PUBLIC SERVANTS can't always offer their clients the help they need, however much they may empathize with them, the deeper question that interests social scientists is whether empathy is meaningfully connected to helping behaviors, and if so, how. The social psychologist C. Daniel Batson wrote more than twenty papers on empathy and conducted multiple studies, mostly with undergraduate students in psychology classes. His most famous theory to come out of all this is called the "empathy-altruism hypothesis," and it claims that empathic concern for another produces altruistic motivation. Because words like "empathy" and "altruism" can have a plethora of meanings, the hypothesis takes a little unpacking.

Empathic concern, Batson says, involves a constellation of feelings including sympathy, compassion, softheartedness, tenderness, sorrow, sadness, upset, distress, concern, and grief. The point is, you feel these things *for* another person, not because his expression is causing you pain. By altruism, Batson means "a motivational state with the ultimate goal of increasing another's welfare." The state is temporary (as opposed to a disposition), and it leads to a specific goal directed entirely toward the other person, irrespective of one's own benefit.

Batson's studies are so important because they supposedly prove that human beings will help each other solely out of the goodness of their hearts. Among the tests he conducted were experiments in which students heard about other students who could no longer come to class because they'd been in a car accident, or who were overwhelmed by the pressures of college. The first set of students felt driven to help. In these experiments, Batson eliminated variables that might be impacting their altruism — such as helping to relieve their own distress, or acting out of social pressure or expectation of reward. He still found, again and again, that people could have a purely altruistic streak.

Batson is not without his detractors. Primary among them is Robert B. Cialdini, a psychology and marketing professor who wrote three bestsellers on the power of persuasion. Cialdini conducted experiments showing that the altruism Batson identifies springs from a perceived *oneness* with another person. In other words, the empathy is driven from a perceived self-other overlap, and the altruistic helping is, in part, directed at the self. Cialdini replicated Batson's experiments but added another step: he had subjects rate how closely they saw themselves in the other. One experiment described a student being evicted from his apartment, for instance, and if the subjects couldn't see themselves in this situation, the helping largely stopped.

This idea seems to track with the HTICs; in addition to empathizing most easily with victims, people extend help to those who mirror them in some way. Children are easy, since we've all been kids, as are those who are explicitly held against their will, since most of us have had some experience of coercion and can imagine a horrific expansion of that. Tougher, perhaps, are the sex workers who aren't instantly resonant — people like B.

Her experience, as a transwoman, is one of fetishization, and she's internalized that. "If some man who ain't my husband or my man wants to have sex with me, then he's going to pay for it," she said. A person like B lies outside the scope of the original vision for the HTIC, and it's not clear she's able to get much benefit from it either.

What B, and many other sex workers, actually need is housing. Eighty-seven percent of street-based prostitutes and forty-three percent of indoor workers in New York City don't have their own stable place to stay. Around 25 percent of the youth who end up at the Covenant House homeless shelter are victims of trafficking or sexual labor. Despite this, the HTICs do not provide emergency housing — only referrals to the same shelters that are notoriously overcrowded already.

Cialdini, along with his colleague Steven L. Neuberg, has argued that empathy only leads to superficial helping. In several experiments, they showed that the empathy-altruism hypothesis isn't relevant to understanding meaningful forms of help. In other words, empathy isn't the route to a substantive solution like housing. When empathy is a prime motivator (as opposed to something more self-serving, like getting praise or avoiding blame), most people will provide help only when it comes at little or no cost to them.

B takes a practical view. She knows housing resources are limited; she knows nobody's going to be able to recognize and meet her particular needs. She feels she has to keep on hustling, and she thinks the mandated counseling is pretty much a waste of her time. She believes everyone would be better served if the court simply ignored people like her and focused instead on the children enslaved to pimps, whom she called "babies getting raped."

WITHIN THE CURRENT SYSTEM, it's nearly impossible to tease apart who's being trafficked and who's doing sex work by choice. Judges don't ask that question, and lawyers typically meet their clients at the moment of their arraignment, which is hardly the time to establish trust. Right up until the judge releases them to their mandated counseling, the defendants have been treated as criminals: they've been arrested, held in a police car and sometimes in a cell, and then brought before a judge. All of this, both Goodman and Bedard assert, is traumatic.

"The existential crisis that I've struggled with for years is the way that people get to us sucks," Goodman said. "But once they're here, good things are happening."

Goodman says she and others have tried to provide services through outreach rather than arrest, but with this route, the real victims of trafficking don't show up. Goodman shook her head. "How else would we connect to this group of people, I just don't know."

The Sex Workers Outreach Project (SWOP) in New York advises police to stop arresting people they assume are being trafficked and instead direct them to safe housing, attorneys, and agencies. But right now, Goodman notes, the relationship between cops and sex workers is too troubled for the police to make such an assertion. During a raid, she says, "everyone will say they're not being trafficked. They're police—and if you don't speak English or you're not here legally, you're peeing your pants, are you kidding? It's so nerve-wracking!"

Goodman's colleagues already piloted something like the SWOP recommendation for adolescents who commit minor crimes. Rather than arresting the kids, police can now send them to diversionary programming and keep them out of court entirely. Unfortunately, it took three years for the DA's office to approve the adolescent program — and prostitution's an even tougher sell.

"People are struggling with a stereotype of trafficking versus who they're actually arresting," Goodman said. "To assume someone who's a victim of sex trafficking is going to be begging for your help and be a quote unquote 'good victim' is never going to happen."

Multiple studies and articles show that sex workers experience harassment or worse at the hands of the police. The most comprehensive and narrative study in New York is over ten years old, but it shows that 30 percent of sex workers report being threatened with violence and 27 percent have actually been assaulted. Five out of thirty were threatened sexually or offered sex to avoid arrest, and one was raped by a cop. A full 77 percent of street-based sex workers have been falsely arrested at some point.

The police can arrest someone on the suspicion of loitering with the intent to commit prostitution; they don't have to witness any solicitation or direct transaction. "Suspicion" can look like anything and, as the advocacy group the Red Umbrella Project intimated in a report, can especially look like racial profiling. The Red Umbrella Project observed over 150 defendants in the Brooklyn HTIC and found that black women made up 65 percent of the cases, in a borough where they only compose 16 percent of the population.

Police in New York, as in many places across the country, have a long and embittered history with many of the communities they protect. While it's been limited lately, there's still a stop-and-frisk law that allows them to search anyone they deem suspicious — a law that has overwhelmingly targeted people of color. This history runs deep; in areas that have been over-incarcerated for generations, there's little trust in law enforcement. Even if each precinct were to undergo sensitivity training on the needs and experiences of sex workers, even if they were all to get on board with the "sex worker as victim" narrative that the new courts are promoting, cops would still have power, and it would be tough to get empathic understanding to flow uphill. It's likely sex workers would still see them as B does when she says, "Cops are just always trying to trap you."

Goodman has tried to shift this dynamic. Since, as she observes, decriminalization of sex work "isn't happening anytime soon," her office has tried to limit the initial harm that the law inflicts. One idea would be to have social service providers actually come along with the police when they do their sweeps or bust brothels, so they could offer women support immediately. So far, though, she says, the agencies aren't interested: they don't want the women to associate their agencies with raids.

In the midtown court, I witnessed only polite exchanges between the defendants and courtroom staff; everything felt brisk and procedural. Goodman says this isn't always the case. If a woman's been held overnight in a cell, for instance, she can be angry, and judges or lawyers can lose patience. Says Goodman, "You see somebody's rap sheet, it's five inches thick; they're coming down off drugs and they're cursing out the court staff—how do you summon up your empathy when that's going on in court?"

In the eighteenth century, Adam Smith warned that "the furious behavior of an angry man is more likely to exasperate us against himself than against his enemies." To ward against getting caught up in the frustration or rage defendants might express in an arrest or court, for instance, Smith wrote, "the spectator must . . . endeavor . . . to put himself in the situation of the other and to bring home to himself every little circumstance of distress which can possibly occur to the sufferer. He must adopt to the whole case of his companion with all its minutest incidents."

Simon Baron-Cohen is a current, prominent voice in empathy research, and he argues that the erosion of such empathy leads, actually, to evil. Baron-Cohen is a professor of developmental psychopathology at the University of Cambridge, and in his book *The*

Science of Evil: On Empathy and the Origins of Cruelty, he dislodges evil from its moral or religious implications and considers it, simply, as objectification. He's echoing Hannah Arendt's idea that evil is a "failure of imagination" and Martin Buber's earlier theories that our existence overall is devalued when we see the other as an object. The point here is that even within an empathically directed project, like these new courts, we can objectify, and when we objectify, the empathy breaks down. And vice versa. The judges, the cops, and the lawyers don't tune in to each new arrest's individual humanity: they're all AP-8s. If it's someone's first arrest, she'll be mandated six sessions; if it's her hundredth, she'll just be mandated more.

Here it can be useful to recall British philosopher Peter Goldie's model for the two primary ways we might put ourselves in the situation of another. One is to imagine what *I* might do in a particular circumstance. The other is to imagine what *she* might do in that circumstance. The latter, he says, is actually impossible. We can't ever know another person's psychology, background, and motivations fully enough to do that. And if we pretend to, we're taking away the other person's agency. So while we're continually embarking on the imaginative project of empathic listening, we're also keeping ourselves in check. An example of this is the way Bedard and Goodman sit back instead of moving forward on a client's behalf when she incriminates her pimp. They can feel for a client, but they can't feel precisely what she needs to do. "We never put any pressure on her, like you need to leave him now or you need to talk to the DA or whatever," Bedard said. "We're just waiting for people's readiness to move forward on those conversations."

It took time, Goodman said, for her to understand what she was seeing in the prostitution courts and what kind of help she could provide. She had worked with trauma and crime survivors and in alternative-to-jail programming for years before she accepted her current position, where, at least in the "pimp-controlled world," there was a "level of rawness" she hadn't seen before. Goodman learned that many of the women and girls who are being trafficked can't or won't leave their pimps right away: they have children with these men, and their extensive arrest history would cause them to lose custody; they fear beatings or even murder; they're addicted to drugs and rely on the men for their supply; they face homelessness, isolation, or any of the innumerable other traumas that any of us would if we left the life we know.

Because of all this, many clients will continue to be arrested again and again. Goodman and her colleagues don't measure success in terms of recidivism as other programs do, but rather by the percentage that maintains some form of contact with the court past their mandated requirement. At this point, it's between 15 and 20 percent. So the team keeps thinking of new ways to put more services in front of the women to utilize when they're ready. Bedard works for a domestic violence prevention program called STEPS, which partners with the court. Through that, they provide childcare and children's therapy. It's also expanded to schools in the city, to reach kids before they get involved in violent relationships. STEPS is one of the few programs, Bedard says, to particularly target young boys, rather than just girls. Overall, one of the most positive outcomes of the HTICs, Goodman thinks, is that the dozen or so agencies that provide for sex workers in New York are working together and coordinating their services.

"People on the ground know all you can work on is engagement and a feeling of safety," she observed. She told me the story of a woman she met five years ago who promised she would never leave her pimp; he was violent; she loved him; they had children together. Goodman didn't push her, but she listened. The other day, this woman called Goodman and said she was ready to get out. Goodman was ready to help her. "It takes people so long to make change."

I find Goodman's value-neutral approach to empathy more useful and effective than a court saddled with an express mission to "give prostitutes an opportunity to get out of the life." After all, even subtle forms of morality can be a major block to empathizing. The philosopher Adam Morton writes about socially repugnant acts, and the ways people will focus on the acts themselves rather than the barriers around those acts. We'll think, "I could never do 'that thing,'" and hence we can't understand the person who did it. If we shift, however, to contemplating whatever rules or morals prohibit "that thing," and the times we may have transgressed similar social objections, our empathy can increase. He writes, "The resemblance to a morally repugnant act lies in the repugnance, rather than the immorality." In other words, we're better off relating to feelings of shame, stigmatization, or isolation than to prostitution itself. And most of us can relate to these: we've been bullied, we've been treated like strangers or transgressors, even if we haven't broken the law. As a queer person, I know these feelings well, but all of us, I think, have been isolated or shamed for our identities or choices in one context or another. A Morton-like empathy allows people to resonate with qualities rather than the crimes, perhaps broadening the scope of inclusion.

Morton also argues that the most empathic approach is to ask "how" rather than "why" someone's come to do the things she's done, especially when situations are morally charged. "How" questions, it seems to me, are particularly beneficial in a place like the HTIC, because they direct the gaze away from the scrutinized women and back to the other part of the equation — the traffickers, the pimps, the johns, and an enormous commercial sex market that makes their work possible. Asking "how" gets us back to something closer to nonviolent communication: the simplest forms of mirroring — before analysis, before judgment — which are, paradoxically, some of the most effective ways to help another person feel seen and heard.

7

Performing Empathy

If we take this back to our communities, I think there'll be a worldwide revolution!"

I was sitting in a rented Brooklyn gallery with some 150 high school students — mostly bused in from nearby (Connecticut, Pennsylvania, the Bronx) but a few dozen had flown all the way from Belfast, Ireland. The event was secular, but the air was charged as though it were a tent revival. The person holding the mic, a black girl from a tony private school in Manhattan, had the fervor of the newly converted. When she said "revolution," everyone cheered.

MC-ing the crowd was Colum McCann, author of *Let the Great World Spin* and president of Narrative 4 (N4), the nonprofit launched in 2013 to promote empathy in teenagers. He stood at the front of the room, the kids and their teachers in a broad horseshoe around him, nearly dancing with excitement. "Yes!" he said to the revolution-girl. "One of the deep problems of the world is that people don't feel listened to." This was the end of the program and all day, attendees had been telling one another individual stories but gushing about the ways this private process could have global implications.

A skinny white boy in a green sweatshirt stood up and said, "This is really beautiful. We're all from different backgrounds, but this shows us we're all human." McCann agreed with this too and spread his arms wide.

"Stories are a form of currency," McCann said. "The more you listen to them, the richer you'll become."

N4 was born, in part, out of tragedy. Shortly after the 2012 Newtown, Connecticut, shootings, a local high school teacher named Lee Keylock invited McCann to his English class to discuss his work. Instead, McCann said, the kids needed to exchange stories about what they'd been through. Afterward, McCann, Keylock, and author Luis Alberto Urrea developed the basic pedagogy for N4, with their tagline, "Fearless hope through radical empathy." Unlike Roots of Empathy with its six-hundred-page book of lesson plans, the N4 "class" is simple and designed to be reproduced by anybody, anywhere. It works like this: two people tell each other a story. Then Person A tells Person B's story back to him (and usually to the group at large) in his own words, as if it happened to him.

"My name is Joanna, and I'm going to tell you a story from when I was twenty-three years old that changed the trajectory of my life," Director of Programs Lee Keylock said from the front of the room, by way of example. The night before, he and his wife had exchanged stories, and they modeled the N4 process by embodying each other for the group. Lee is in his early forties, sandy-haired and British, and his wife, Joanna, is American, with an open face and long hair with bangs. Joanna seemed nervous. Lee went on to tell about the way, he (she) left a husband-to-be after seeing *Thelma and Louise*. "I saw my life flash in front of my eyes," he said, helplessly tossing his hands upward. "We had bridesmaids, and a huge wedding planned . . . I told him we're not getting married."

Joanna flipped the process, saying her name was Lee and she was born in an old English town with castles and a river. She didn't try to mimic the British accent or Lee's gestures, but the effect was mesmerizing. She was searching, in the telling, to get some essential element of Lee's story just right. It was this reach that was so moving —and also the way Lee's eyes clouded and turned inward; he was feeling his own experience through the mouth of another.

After the demonstration, Keylock and McCann broke the room up into groups of fifteen to twenty, which then paired off to tell each other their stories in private. Kids were coupled with adults, students who had flown in from Ireland told stories to teenagers from the South Bronx. Some took notes. Others just gazed into space, absorbing, nodding intently. When the small groups reconvened, the teenagers, at least, seemed changed. Gone were the coltish girls with long brushed manes who kicked at the floor toward the few boys (girls outnumbered them four to one) in the flirty mating dance of the early morning. Gone were the slouchy boys in oversized jeans who shrugged back at them. In their place were sixteen human beings, sitting upright and alert.

"My name is Meghan Edwards," said a boy in a checkered shirt solemnly. He glanced at his phone for notes. "And this is the story of a time I lost my mittens."

This first story was simple, about the shame and pain of a little, seemingly negligible loss, but other stories were bigger. One person told of being mugged, another of the family breakup after the dad couldn't stop drinking. One lanky Brooklyn boy talked about his lifelong goal to be the top girl's clog dancer in Ireland — and nobody laughed, such was the totality of his transformation. Without fail, the person whose story was being told would look down at first, remembering, and then tip her head back up, one ear slightly lifted, eyes at that middle distance, caught somewhere between self and not-self.

"It's amazing, hearing yourself from somebody else," one girl said in the wrap-up discussion, and everybody nodded. Another added, "But I sound so vulnerable and unsure. I wonder if I really sound that way."

The kids were clearly hungry for, and sated by, this reflection of themselves, and I questioned whether this was merely an extension of the social media universe they all swam in, or a contradiction of it. All the kids I know post highly curated stories of themselves everywhere, constantly, online, and live for the thousand "likes"; perhaps N4 was replicating this rapt audience in real time. Or maybe it was doing something different.

"This can bridge disparities in social and economic groups," said Martha Rosario, a girl from a public school in the South Bronx with whom I spoke after the session. Martha had already been through an N4 storytelling day—with a group of teenagers from a private school in Riverdale, the upscale side of the Bronx. In a way, even online, you're keeping to your same social networks, and because so much of what you post, and read, is fantasy, you don't really know what even your close neighbors are like. For instance, Martha had heard the kids from Riverdale were served their lunches by private chefs in a lunchroom as grand as Hogwarts. When the Riverdale kids showed up for N4, Martha had her defenses up.

"I thought they'd be put off by our small school, that they'd be presumptuous and pompous, and not street smart like us," she said. But then they swapped stories and found their struggles— with school, with parents, with sports coaches—shockingly simi- lar. "When we were able to see they're not just these rich kids, then the size of the room just faded into the background. Nobody cared about the schools. We were just having conversation."

Still, I noticed throughout the day that the types of conversations that teenagers and adults were having were distinctly different. No matter the harrowing content—dad leaving, someone dying—if a kid told the story, it ended on a happy note. "Now everything's fine; my family is closer than ever" seemed to be the culminating phrase to most exchanges, and I wondered if this was perhaps the echo of an online culture intent on only the shiniest of self-productions. Or maybe the kids were still steeped in five-paragraph-essay mode and felt compelled to tie up messy lives with a trite thesis. In any case, the adults' stories were more nuanced, more loose and unspooling—I heard patchwork, free-associative accounts of race awareness, or the cumulative effect of micro-aggressions, without the same compulsion to tie up or conclude. A major tenet of N4 is to avoid prompts; participants are encouraged to tell whatever story they like, but I wonder if this can also encourage a kind of packaged performance rather than the true vulnerability the kids seemed to feel they were exchanging.

Still, another tenet of N4 is its simplicity and flexibility. Unlike curricula designed only for trained practitioners to employ, N4 was created for anyone to export. And adapt to their needs. If I tried this with my students, I thought, I'd add a prompt. "Now that you know the power of this, you can do it in other communities, you can do it on Skype," Colum McCann crowed from the front of the room, like a preacher priming his flock. "They do brain images, and when your brain is telling someone else's story it's like a carnival in there. You're being creative and you're shaping the future!"

While there's certainly something off-putting in the Pollyanna-ish quality of such overly grand promises, there may be a reason the leaders of empathy movements carry proselytizers' zeal: we need it. If modernity stripped us of collective, binding religion, what is left to make us collectively, bindingly moral? Philosopher and sociologist Eva Illouz writes that religion gave us our saints and our stories—the beautifying features that made life bearable. While modernity privileged the individual and stripped us of our blinders to manmade cruelties, it also stripped us of our stories. Empathy, as a concept, gives us back all three: a moral, a story, and a tie between us all. This could be one more clue to its promise and its hold.

IF THERE'S ONE MAN for whom empathy is a near-religious mission, it's Edwin Rutsch. Rutsch has conducted and uploaded more than three hundred interviews with empathy experts onto his "Culture of Empathy" website. The name denotes the global phenomenon he's trying to foster. I met him at his hundred-year-old house in El Cerrito, California, where he runs the site; stores an "empathy tent," which he regularly sets up outside the Berkeley subway station for passersby who want to give or receive empathy; and is working on a pilot for an empathy reality show.

"I sometimes feel a bit alone," Rutsch admitted, from what he called "empathy headquarters," a tidy home office with three desks, a mocha-colored futon, and the same two dozen or so books on empathy that I have on my shelves. "I have twenty-two thousand people on the empathy page on Facebook, but I'll go out and do an empathy tent and nobody shows up."

Rutsch isn't giving up, though. He's an earnest man in his early fifties, with an earnest face: blue eyes behind wire-rimmed glasses; thin, black hair tied into a low ponytail; and an easy, slightly bucked smile. He considers himself a "focal point for the empathy movement," and his basic mission is to be a repository and a hub for new research and dialogues about empathy, and to provide evidence of empathy in real time for as wide an audience as he can muster. His proposed family empathy reality show is an example of this.

"The *Supernanny* show [in the United States and United Kingdom] had more than four or five million viewers, so people want to see things modeled in action," he said. Rutsch is currently inspired by a trend called empathic design: businesses interview consumers to incorporate their lifestyles, needs, problems, and even latent wishes into the design of a product. "We apply this process to designing more empathy in families. Say we interview a family to find out where the problem area is, and then we go into creativity mode where we're brainstorming with the team, and all kinds of ideas come up. And then you kind of home in on which idea you want to work on, like a prototype," Rutsch said, explaining that agreeing on a plan of action is a kind of empathy in itself. "Then you test it and you test it again, and the testing is like empathizing, asking what's working, what's not working."

Despite Rutsch's process-oriented approach, I was concerned that he, like so many other well-intentioned empathy preachers, was sipping his inspiration from the capitalist brew we're all swimming in, which guides us to an end product, a result, something to buy. This parasitic model of empathy is a loop: corporations serve our needs and whims to serve their pockets and call it empathy, and then, primed for such exchange, we're ready to worship at empathy's altar, uncritically, ready to be served again.

But Rutsch made a distinction between empathy types. Yes, he admitted, there is a ubiquitous consumerist empathy based first on assessment and then giving to get, but Rutsch calls this transactional empathy, a sort of one-to-one equation. Rutsch is more interested in what he calls transformative empathy, which changes both parties entirely. He says transformative empathy works like this:

"It's a whole arc of experiences. First there's self-empathy, which is feeling into your own experience; and then cognitive empathy, feeling into the other's experience and creating an understanding, like a cognitive map of who they are, and maybe having inferences and having a sense of their intentions and all of that; then there's what I call imaginative empathy, which is the role-playing part, so I can take on you [in my mind], maybe I can say what is it like to be you?" For Rutsch, there's a constant interplay between imagining the other and feeling one's own experience. "I feel into myself and imagine that role-playing. And then there's the empathic creativity or action, which is where we really connect with each other; we work together and there's a creativity where we go forward. That's the transformational empathy."

Rutsch envisions this kind of exchange not just interpersonally or within families but on a national stage. "I'm moving away from saying I'm progressive to saying I'm in the empathy party movement," Rutsch said. "We need a separate and clear movement that's to support empathy for progressives and conservatives, and bringing them together."

Rutsch actually launched his work on the heels of the Obama inauguration, after the president spoke repeatedly of the nation's empathy deficit during his campaign. After Obama was elected, Obama for America — the group that sought to mobilize supporters around his legislative agenda — held meetings in the East Bay. Rutsch expected to mobilize around empathy. "I asked the person in charge if she would do an interview with me about empathy, and she said she didn't have time. Somehow Obama's rhetoric didn't get integrated into the machinery of the campaign," Rutsch noted, explaining that Obama for America was focused entirely on healthcare and the war, the "typical talking points." Rutsch lamented the way progressives can't articulate and defend their values the way conservatives do, and that empathy could be an organizing principle. "If you just list all the times Obama talked about empathy, I don't understand why he didn't put together an empathy team."

For Rutsch, empathy isn't an abstraction like hope or kindness but rather a strategy for action, a way of seeing through. He leads empathy circles for people in conflict, and he imagines implementing this process in the public sphere too. In empathy circles, "you use reflective listening and turn talking, where I reflect back what you've said until you feel fully heard, and you reflect back what I said and we go back and forth like that," Rutsch explained. "This structures a dialogue to take it out of conflict and into empathy."

Once people experience this kind of empathy, in his tent or in a circle, or witness it on a TV show, Rutsch hopes they'll be on board to "build a movement to have empathy be a primary social value. How do we design societally and structurally around it?"

One example, he said, might be our court system. I knew this: I'd been exploring the notion of empathy in the judicial process exhaustively. But Rutsch broke it down: "There's a jury and a judge and defendant and plaintiff and they're put into a sort of battle arena and through this battle we're going to come to the truth," Rutsch said. But if we changed the premise from a battle to a dialogue, then the notion of bias wouldn't even factor. If we instead saw everyone in the courtroom as interconnected, with each person's actions and

speech affecting the whole, then empathy would become an imperative. "The notion of bias comes within a premise of judgment and
disconnection, and so when you get past those premises, it's a whole
different paradigm."

I left Rutsch's house, with the poppies and bougainvillea trailing
sweetly in his yard, thinking I was glad to have him and his utopian
visions in the world. But I also wasn't surprised this vision didn't
get much traction. It's not just that empathy is squirrelly, too slippery and broad, to grip as a social mission. There's also something
suffocating and coopting about being forced to empathize in some
new world order. I want to hold on to my defenses and edges, my
resistance to look; I can't be open to a pervasive "you" all the time,
my intuition cries, or an inner "I" could break apart. And maybe
this is why empathy, at times, feels treacly and oppressive, or even a
bit embarrassing: there are things in the other, we know, we cannot
even begin to imagine. We don't even want to try.

I'm referring mainly to trauma, of the very type we see in politics
and courtrooms, with their wars and their crimes, and their victims
of both. If we approach this work entirely through an empathy lens,
we not only run the risk of ritualized secondary traumatization and
trauma fatigue but also repeat misrecognition. Elie Wiesel said the
Greeks invented tragedy, the Renaissance the sonnet, and our generation the literature of testimony. Memoir, documentary film, the
proliferation and range of journalistic dispatches, all speak to a collective urge to bear witness in a post-Holocaust age. And perhaps
the rise in a call for empathy is a collective urge to respond. But
Primo Levi, maybe the greatest or most urgent and prolific Holocaust writer of all, said, "The intrinsic horror of this human con-
dition has imposed a sort of reserve on all the testimony." By this
I think he meant that human beings will react to human horror
with a softening narrative; we will pocket ourselves into assurances
of "never again" or delude ourselves with fantasies of sympathetic

alignment. To paraphrase the poet Paul Celan, there isn't anybody to bear witness for the witness, and I think there's truth to that: in real horror, we may want empathy, but as in death, we are alone.

And still, the better option is quieter than the imaginative leaps and pulls of empathy. The better option is a kind of stillness, a being beside, without always seeking an inner resonance, because sometimes there's none to be had.

In other words, empathy has its place, but it isn't every place. When I met with Rutsch, he asked me many questions about my own family; he did this because he used his own family as an example of an empathy circle in action and because he's a good listener and wanted to exchange. Rutsch's story was about a Christmas visit with his family of origin. In this story, Rutsch's mother and sister-in-law got into an argument about hiding the presents well enough so the kids couldn't dig into them. Rutsch held an empathy circle, unpeeling layers of misunderstanding until the sister-in-law finally revealed she had never really felt she was part of the family. Once the mother could hear this core pain, and reassure her, the issue of the presents evaporated.

This was a happy story with a happy ending, and in the face of it, I shut down. When empathy is the stated goal or frame for a particular kind of telling, then the teller tries to match his environment in a kind of empathic hum. I think of the tightly packaged stories the kids told at Narrative 4 in an effort to be easily identified and arranged in the mind of another. My family stories don't have happy endings or even endings, really; they're studded with cliffhangers and sharp turns, incest, abandonment, and abuse that goes back generations. I don't tell these stories very often, for the discomfort they evoke and for the way, when I feel the listener's empathy rise up around me like a smoke, I choke and sputter my way deeper into an internal isolation. Some memories haven't settled their way into understanding, and another's empathy can feel foreclosing of my own search for meaning. When I talk about my own crises, I don't believe in empathy's reach, even when someone can find an aspect of my experience to match their own, or imagine their way into my head. To be more true: I don't want empathy—to be met or seen or understood or, even worse, transformed. I want rather a carefully mediated space that says I can bear witness to my own trials without invasion, that I can be alone as I'll always be, with others simply there.

There's a kind of theater that hits this form of empathy, that mediates between this wish for pure bearing witness and the other, outsized, longing to connect. It's called Playback Theatre, and it's a kind of dramatic improvisation in which audience members tell stories and see them immediately replayed, live, by the troupe. There are sixty Playback companies internationally and nearly fifty in the United States. My best friend, Teresa Dias, is a Playback actor with True Story Theater, a company in Boston, and she explained it like this: "This is a forum where you can have a hard conversation, where you can chew on a theme that's uncomfortable, that gets you in trouble, that gets you into arguments with people." But in her next breath she made a turn: "This is a place for two hours where you can tell your own personal experience and be seen and be heard and be held in a really generous way."

I first heard of Playback eight years ago when Teresa joined the company, and I thought it sounded risky. The shows' themes were things like racism, disability, socioeconomics, shame, and death, and the idea of five actors inviting a stranger to share a story from those hot waters risked getting somebody burned in the artistic reinterpretation. But no, she said, invariably the teller gained some insight on his experience, usually because the actors replayed some core truth they intuited but that he hadn't shared directly. The actors won't project the story into the future at all, but they will flesh out characters the teller may have only lightly sketched. "How did you know my brother was mad?" the teller will gasp, astonished, after his story's been performed. And sometimes the actors won't entirely know themselves.

"Improvisation is a lightning bolt. All theater is a creative act, but improvisation is instant. People talk about channeling and being in a zone and all these things—there's something about improvisation that is a pure type of inspiration," Teresa said. In Playback rehearsal, the actors work primarily on deep listening—for the plot points and organization of a story but also for broader social themes and undercurrents of emotional truth that the teller might be expressing through gesture or tone, if not in language. "There are a lot of these magical threads that come together where people say, 'How did you know that?' or 'How did you guys communicate with each other?'"

Good Playback Theatre is strong ensemble work; actors will step into set roles without even making eye contact with one another, as they seem to know where they'll fit naturally. Teresa says this is called "tele," meaning empathetic resonance or understanding without words. When tele unites the actors, it also unites the audience in a collective, larger-than-life experience. She likened the whole of Playback Theatre to the San Francisco earthquake of 1989. Teresa and I had been sunbathing on her rooftop when the earthquake struck; one moment we were blissfully soaking up rays; the next, the electrical wires were swinging loose and we were crab-crawling our way over the pitched and roiling roof back to the open window. In an instant, without speaking, we were out on the street.

"Everybody was like, 'Who needs batteries?' and 'Do you have a radio?' There was a connectedness because all of us just experienced this earthquake, and you're going to reach out to your fellow man. I feel that when an audience sees a show—there's a common thread that's amplified," Teresa said. The storytelling an audience member does, in other words, is the earthquake, a shared traumatic event. It's what happens after that elevates it: the theatrical interpretation inspires caring and connectedness that give the trauma meaning and perspective.

I went to a Playback show recently in the small Boston suburb of Arlington. Nestled next to Cambridge, Arlington is middle-class and white; the middle-aged audience, in their wire-rim glasses and soft fleece hoodies, reflected that demographic. The theme for the show was stigma. The show was held in a yoga studio where rent was cheap. Forty-five audience members shuffled to their folding chairs in their socks. At the front of the room were four cubes the size of milk crates and a clothing rack draped in jewel-colored scarves. Two musicians played hand drums at a table scattered with kazoos, chimes, and Tibetan singing bowls. After four actors in black took their place at the cubes, a woman named Anne Ellinger addressed the crowd. She would be that night's "conductor," a staple role in Playback Theatre.

"Who would think a room full of people would come out on a Saturday night to talk about stigma?" she asked, smiling, her arms loose at her side. Anne is fifty-nine, with tight grey curls and a broad smile. She asked the group to call out types of stigma they'd experienced and the room erupted with words: age, disability, gender identity, religion, adult illiteracy. She then asked someone to share simply how she was feeling right then.

A woman in her sixties answered: "I feel nervous about being here because something might come up and yet I know I need to be here." This was the first opportunity for the Playback actors to reflect an experience, and they did it with a technique they call "fluid sculpture." One actor came forward, raising his hands and looking up toward the sky, claiming, "I feel nervous" on repeat. Another, slightly more sinister, sidled up next to him and ran one arm up between his, pointing her finger sharply and growling, "Something might come up!" Another actor brought his cube to stand above them both, arms draped protectively around them to soothe, "I know I need to be here." The woman in the audience smiled in recognition: yes, this was exactly how she felt.

The next stories were harder and more complex. At the actors' disposal are several types of theatrical possibilities, called "forms." Sometimes they replay a story using only song and movement, the central ideas abstracted into gestures, expressions, and jumps. Sometimes, in a form called a chorus, each actor will play the teller, mining different aspects of the experience. Other times the replay will be more concrete, with actors casting themselves directly into the roles outlined in a story, but in this case, an actor might swoop in as an unseen but powerful force, like racism or generational poverty. The conductor calls out the form before each act, but other than that, everything is spontaneously born on the spot.

"How about 'Song and Movement,'" Anne the conductor said, after a sad woman with long grey hair and glasses told a story in which she herself was the stigmatizer: she had harshly ostracized her daughter's wife and now regretted it. But the daughter and her partner didn't want her back in their lives.

In the reenactment, Teresa played the mother and a man named Brandon played the stigmatized couple; the other two actors went to the side to sing. Somehow, it wasn't much of a leap for a young black man to play both members of the lesbian couple: for one thing, the teller's longing seemed directed at a unified entity, and splitting that target into two bodies would have hit a literal truth but not an emotional one. And second, when Brandon danced, he *was* a proud, rejected couple; he splayed his arms in rage and resistance, and then curled them round himself, two parts of a whole.

The musician at the table thumped a frame drum in a heartbeat rhythm, while a blonde singer let out a moan that rose to a wail. Teresa, playing the mother, marched across the stage to the beat, her arms waving. Teresa now works as an arts therapist but she used to be a professional aerialist, and that sinewy strength is still present. She grabbed a scarf from the rack, faced her daughters (i.e., Brandon) like a storm, and hurled the scarf at his chest. He held it like the toxic bundle it was, away from him, disgusted, while the two singers had found a joint melody. They were singing, in a round, lines of "echoing the pain" and "can't take it back." Teresa had moved to the corner of the room, shock and horror on her face. Brandon followed her there with the scarf and dropped it at her feet. Teresa picked it up gingerly—now the scarf was a snake—as the singers sang, "I'm trying, I'm trying," and "Please forgive my injury." Teresa crumpled the snake into a ball and buried her face there, shoulders shaking.

In every performance, the teller watches the replay from a special seat at the side of the stage so the audience can watch her watching her story unfold. This time, there was a kind of dazed recognition drifting across the woman's face in waves; she seemed almost hypnotized. But in the audience, I happened to be sitting next to her husband. He was openly weeping as Teresa approached Brandon one more time with the crumpled-up scarf. Brandon wouldn't take it, though his face was mournful as he shifted his body away from hers, his chin lifted with tentative, lonely pride. Teresa glanced back down at the scarf and reluctantly held it to her own abdomen, as though it were her burden to keep, and leaned her head on the shoulder of her symbolic daughters. As if on cue, the music stopped, Teresa closed her eyes, and the lights went down.

I was surprised to realize later that the lights hadn't actually gone down. We were in a yoga studio with a flip switch and nobody was stationed there. But the piece had felt so complete, so practiced and contained, that I had forgotten it was improvised. "When it works it's gorgeous," Teresa said. Even though the woman hadn't made amends with her daughter, the subtext was that she clearly wanted to, and ending on a gesture of tentative reconciliation was both empathic and good storytelling: it moved the piece beyond its first iteration. When it was over, the woman was almost speechless but obviously moved. But sometimes, Teresa said, the troupe will overstep and a teller will say he feels misunderstood.

"And then we will do an ending all over again," Anne told me. I met with Anne and Christopher, Anne's husband and the company director, at their home the next morning to eat croissants and talk Playback. Their house was easy to spot: it was bright orange in a row of whites and greys, bedecked with a wooden sign that read "Wildest Dreams." They're both fifty-nine, have been partners for over thirty years, and regularly filled in each other's answers.

"The key of what we're trying to do is to model good communication, and good communication doesn't happen without full feedback," Christopher said. He was one of the singers when Brandon and Teresa danced, but throughout the evening, he played the "costume of skin," a father, the voice of India, and a young girl forced to diet. "It's not about us showing how brilliant we are. It's about us being willing to humbly say, 'We're doing our best to hear you and we won't always get it. Please tell us what your truth is.'"

One thing the company won't play back is the precise words or actions of someone's trauma; they're very careful not to retraumatize through direct replica. So if someone tells the story of being called names, for instance, an actor might fiercely shout gibberish across the stage. Teresa told me that once, during the reenactment of a murder someone witnessed, the company performed a scene in slow motion to make the impact more abstract and diffuse while still true.

"If it's in slow motion, it's metaphorized," Anne explained. "We're focusing much more on the inner experience than the outer experience."

Plus, she said, the mission of the company is "social healing through theater," so it's important not to leave the teller, or the audience, suspended only in their pain. Anne, or another conductor, will often ask a teller about his resources, or what sustains him through whatever difficult story he's told. Anne's email tagline is "Creating a culture of empathy, respect, and creativity," and I wondered whether it was really empathic to push her audience toward a happy ending when perhaps there wasn't one.

"It's not about the happy ending," she replied. "If we only show the painful part it ends up not feeling reflective of their life because none of us are only our challenges. And people are helped by seeing this: 'Here you are. You're still alive.'"

Throughout the prior evening's performance, Anne asked the audience for quick responses to what they were seeing, what they were feeling. She did this again and again. Nobody commented on the reinterpretations or the artistic modifications to the stories. Rather, what they repeated, over and over, was that the actors *listened* to them. "What was stirred up for me was the generous listening," someone said. And then, "There wasn't judgment—it was just listening." And—"You were getting in one person's skin and listening."

There's a difference between what feels like mere listening and what is actually an interpretation—and in this way, this theatrical empathy is something like therapy. We like to feel that the major revelations in a therapeutic setting are our own, when in reality, we're often guided there, quite pointedly. It's not surprising that Playback has one of its main roots in psychodrama. Launched in 1975 by husband-and-wife team Jonathan Fox and Jo Salas, Playback is different from psychodrama in that it has an audience and utilizes real actors. In psychodrama, a licensed psychodramatist helps a patient through a conflict by directing a small group of people to act out the dynamic before him. Fox was trained in this method but wanted to expand the concept both theatrically and across a broader spectrum of social stories.

Anne and Christopher launched their company in 2001 after a couple of out-of-state Playback troupes performed at conferences for the other business they cofounded, a nonprofit dedicated to encouraging bolder donations to charities. Because they were already comfortable talking with people about the touchy subject of money and class difference, they were eager to jump into fraught territory with Playback: they pulled actors from an improv group Christopher was in, and their first show was about AIDS and September 11.

Recently Christopher brought in new actors for the now twenty-four-member company. While the actors have been mostly volunteers over the company's life, both Teresa and Christopher say they benefit personally from performing the stories. "The level of greater openness and empathy and compassion I have for other people, and the way I'm more aware when I'm starting to label or judge people different from me and releasing that, has been quite profound," Christopher said of his time performing.

In one of the few books about Playback, the originator Jo Salas writes about the way the chaos of experience is redeemed when it is transmuted into a story. The formal elements—a rising plotline, a climax, a conclusion—all hemmed in by themes and cultural contexts, make meaning of otherwise random or cruel occurrences. That's why, of course, we're hungry for storytelling and why the kids in Narrative 4, who have less experience, narrativize their lives with such tidy endings. And I'm like anyone: I love stories. I tell them for a living. But I also know, perhaps because of this work, what gets foreclosed when you polish some facts to a high sheen and ignore others for the sake of arc and plot: a kind of grand mythology can trump the quieter but also rich and potentially useful confusion of life as it's lived. There's a faint line, in other words, between imposing meaning and reflecting, and both empathy and Playback are most powerful when they harness the latter.

Then again, for Christopher, empathy is a means to his higher goal, which is social healing. Storytelling can sometimes forecast a path. In one study of forty-seven adults who wrote personal narratives alongside their twelve sessions of talk therapy, increased agency appeared in the stories *before* their mental health improved.

And so, while we may not all engage in the kinds of narrativizing group activities of N4 and Playback Theatre, we can think about sorting our lives into stories, and about being more cognizant of the kinds of listening-repeating approach that these groups represent in our day-to-day interactions. Through this, perhaps, we can grow more curious about one another. And we can think sometimes in metaphor, as a kind of bridge, when the concrete stories don't reach the edges of shared experience.

In the last act of the night, the Playback Theatre performed my favorite piece, and it didn't involve a story at all. Anne asked five audience members to call out a feeling or experience they had watching the show. Five actors formed a V onstage, and one by one they stepped into the V's point, acting out the prompts. Teresa's came from an older woman who said, "Every life has value." Teresa bent from the waist and mimed plucking a dandelion. She brought it to her lips and blew.

PART III

Forgiveness

8

Fall from the Tree

When I began this book project, I knew I would have to venture into a territory I found particularly distasteful — a realm I had an almost knee-jerk negative reaction to. It's a category of empathy around which a whole industry is now cranking. I just didn't know how deeply I would have to enter it, and for what reasons.

This branch of the empathy tree is self-empathy, and the fruit it bears is forgiveness, both for oneself and for others. Essentially, the thinking goes, forgiveness is a self-serving act, as carrying around anger and resentment only hurts the self. So one needs a healthy dose of self-empathy to merit even the desire to forgive another. But I felt self-empathy smacked of narcissism. Self-empathy was code for selfish, one more link in a long chain of American entitlement.

I didn't buy the line — preached explicitly or implicitly by Nonviolent Communication, twelve-step groups, or any of the other large-scale peace and recovery movements, and already practiced by thousands — that in order to have empathy for others you have to first have empathy for yourself. To me, this sounded like indulgent, self-help mush, akin to taking a bubble bath when your child is hungry.

Besides, I didn't know what it meant, self-empathy. How could one step outside her skin and administer first aid? It seemed hokey, forced, or childish. I wanted to get on to the *real* empathy, the difficult empathy: the empathizing with enemies or psychopaths or impossible others.

I didn't want to climb out onto that branch and explore it, but as I pushed further into this book project, I realized I would have to. This third section moves beyond small-scale empathy practiced between individuals, or even the variations that emerge in court-rooms and classrooms, and into the kind that people muster for those who have committed gross crimes against humanity. And I found this kind of empathy, by definition, flows in two directions at once: people who practice it must both humanize an outsize, ste-reotyped "other," often dubbed as evil, and they must dig deep per-sonally, enacting a psychic self-care to protect themselves from such potential danger.

IN THE UNITED STATES, the biggest, most commercialized kind of self-empathy is something called "mindful self-compas-sion." Mindfulness is its own practice, born of a Western approach to Buddhism and popularized by Jon Kabat-Zinn, with his eight-week courses in stress reduction and the quiet mind. There are now nearly a thousand certified mindfulness instructors located in ev-ery state and more than thirty countries. A friend suggested I take an online version of the Kabat-Zinn course when I was at a par-ticularly low point in my relationship with Seth, and mindfulness, as I experienced it through this particular class, is a way of using meditation to create space among thoughts, feelings, and ingrained reactions. Teachers guide you through sitting and movement and eating meditations to help you notice the feelings that arise in the body, and learn to watch the feelings shift, without judgment, rather than reacting to them. This, over time, helps a person to slow down and recognize that he has some choice in his responses. Compassion comes in when we can witness our suffering in this sort of detached, observant state (rather than simply reacting to it or trying to fix it without awareness), and when we can extend that compassion to others who are suffering too.

Major institutes and universities have devoted themselves to the study of compassion in the last few decades; among them are Stanford's Center for Compassion and Altruism Research and Education, Berkeley's Greater Good Science Center, and UC San Diego's Center for Empathy and Compassion. Although compassion's definition can vary as widely as empathy's, they're correlates. And mindful *self*-compassion (MSC) is the newest bird in the nest. Based structurally on the Kabat-Zinn classes, but with more focus on training the compassion inward, MSC was developed in 2010 and has now been taught to six hundred instructors, who teach it all over the world.

When I first heard about it, I imagined anyone who indulged in the practice to be precisely that: indulgent. I pictured self-loving hippie types who exuded self-righteous elitism. They couldn't find anything bigger or more important to direct their compassion toward than the almighty self? I obviously was just a little judgmental, and besides I had some research to do. I decided to jump right in: I signed up for a weekend intensive course in MSC.

It turned out the 150 or so attendees were also squirmy, also judging, also, like me, a little scared. The MSC conference was held on the Harvard campus, sponsored by Cambridge Health Alliance and Harvard Medical School's Center for Mindfulness and Compassion. The group primarily was made up of therapists — we were there to learn about the way mindful self-compassion could intersect with another, more established psychological method called Internal Family Systems, and most of the attendees had some footing in one training or the other. They didn't look like hippies, but they were mostly older white women, with soft grey haircuts and swirly silver earrings, shouldering canvas tote bags from public-radio pledge drives. It was a uniform look. Still, when Chris Germer, a founder of MSC, asked the audience to call out preconceived notions about the practice, the response, and resistance, were robust.

"It's selfish."

"Indulgent."

"Pollyannaish, sugarcoating."

"An excuse for non-action."

People from all over the room mirrored my own misgivings about self-compassion. Germer, who is tall and a little shy in front of groups and so speaks haltingly, countered with research that showed that people who regularly practice MSC are more likely to engage in perspective-taking, are more caring and supportive in romantic relationships, and are more likely to compromise and seek collaborative solutions. Self-compassion, in other words, allowed for more intake of the other. He then went on to define the difference between empathy and compassion.

"Carl Rogers defines empathy as an accurate understanding of another's world as seen from the inside," Germer said, invoking the humanistic psychologist. "Empathy is where really we feel a sense almost identical to a person outside. Compassion is a deep feeling for the suffering of others, plus the wish and effort to alleviate the suffering."

Germer then went on to claim that empathy and compassion actually utilize entirely different neural pathways: in fMRI scans, compassion lights up the medial orbital frontal cortex, which Germer called "a neural network of positive emotions." When people were told to empathize, the insula and middle syndrome cortex lit up, which he said correlated to negative feelings. "Basically," he continued, "when somebody is suffering and we feel empathy, parts of our brain that are suffering get activated. Yet, when we see the same suffering activated with compassion, our brain shows positive affect."

The reason, he said, is the kindness. With empathy, we're "trapped" in simply sharing someone else's affect, but compassion offers an escape valve, because we wish to improve the situation.

I wasn't so sure about this construction, especially as empathy, in many common understandings, does have a prosocial component embedded within it. Germer was also indulging in a bit of name-calling himself, insisting that compassion was inherently better than empathy. He said that people often complained of compassion fatigue but what they really meant was that they had empathy fatigue —they felt too much, too frequently, the pull of others' emotions, without the relief of *doing* anything about it. The simple act of wishing to alleviate another's suffering, the cornerstone of compassion, alleviates the fatigue of feeling their pain. And tending to one's own suffering first, the mindful self-compassion, opens the gates for tending to others.

He led us in an exercise. We were all sitting in a barrel-shaped room, all concrete and windows draped in filmy grey curtains, facing forward in metal folding chairs. Germer asked us to get comfortable, to close our eyes. He said that if any of us wanted to leave this room, we could, adding that sometimes the most self-compassionate thing was avoidance. He said that a history of trauma often made self-compassion too confrontational. As he asked us to remember an incident from our past that was embarrassing but not utterly shameful (about a three on a scale of ten), people started shifting in their seats. When he told us to really drop into this memory, to feel it in our bodies and then to physically touch a part of ourselves—say, put a hand on our own heart—a few people stood up. The woman next to me noisily gathered her things and walked out. This self-compassion was *hard*.

I remembered a fairly benign incident from thirty years back, from a time in high school when an older boy mocked me in front of other kids. It's the kind of memory that still causes me to flush a little in the retelling, but I can tell it out loud and laugh at myself. When I related the story to my best friend after the conference, she didn't laugh: she frowned sympathetically and said, "Awww." This is exactly the sound Germer asked us to make for ourselves, out loud, as we continued to dwell in our memories. A few more people got up. It felt cheesy, sure, cooing for myself over a distant and minor slight, but I could stay with it: I was in a room with a hundred-plus others doing the same thing. I wanted to try. As we moved on from cooing and touching to smiling at the internal image of our younger selves, my self-consciousness shifted to something softer and my embarrassment did too. I felt lighter in general, and more tender toward the scene in high school, toward the boy who caused it and toward myself.

This was obviously self-compassion-lite—a quickie exercise to help us touch what could be possible with deeper work. Although I felt less squeamish about MSC in general, I still couldn't see myself signing up for an eight-week course. But I also didn't know how much, in the course of writing this book, my life would change. For the worse.

This is what happened: Before Seth began his transition, he told me that if the hormones affected our relationship negatively in any way, he would stop. I knew this promise would come to haunt me because it wasn't really his to make. I knew that the person before me would change foundationally, like a clock rearranging its gears that later wouldn't know it used to forecast time. He might remember saying the words, but he wouldn't remember being the person who could say them. I knew this, even then, with a prescience that frightened me.

Even so, I nurtured him through the long years when he oscillated between states of terror over altering the way he would look and be looked upon, and fury that we lived in a world that forced such a choice. I changed his drains and took pictures when he finally and proudly had top surgery six years ago. I talked him through the first time he wore a man's swimsuit at the pool and watched him from the bleachers. I argued with confused border agents at airports when passports didn't match presentation and Seth was pulled to the scary little room with only one chair. When he was ready, but utterly overwhelmed, I found the kind doctor upstate who would take down his history and prescribe him his testosterone. I gave Seth his very first shot in her office.

I did this because I saw, as Seth saw, burning brightly beneath both of our fears, the person Seth needed to become. This, I think, is love. Our fears of course were different. Seth is a psychologist and was afraid he would lose his practice, that his patients would all run away. He was afraid he wouldn't like the changes, so fast and so permanent, that telltale voice, the potential balding. I was afraid, really, only of losing Seth, that the chemical swirl of hormones would tip his heart away from mine. If I gave this fear words at the time, I would have said that I was scared he'd suddenly want men, because that's the story that's out there, circulating like a schoolyard taunt. But then Seth, my Seth, more than anything, was afraid of regret, terrified of dying in a cloud of what if, of his real life left unlived. I cherished Seth more than my fears; I had to help him be more alive.

For the first six months, I gave Seth his weekly shots; he was also afraid of needles. I made recordings of his changing voice so he would have a chronicle of his journey. I took notes at the doctor's appointments. I researched name-change processes, found lawyers, made files. I was transition's secretary, treasured and indispensable. I told myself this was empathy, meeting Seth's needs before he knew he had them, but really it was terror of being deemed unnecessary now that the process was truly underway. When, one day, Seth took his syringes into his own hands, I was bereft.

And then came other signs, scarier ones. He started to say he was "ambivalent" about our relationship. He spoke about a dynamic in our exchanges, one he said had always been there, that I had seen, though not as starkly. We knew each other so well, could predict each shift in mood and preempt downturns with gentle humor or pleas to connect. Seth called this dynamic merging, and suddenly, on testosterone, he didn't want it anymore. This dynamic, he said, in all its empathy, was smothering.

Seth wanted to become his own person, but, through my eyes, this person was bitter, sullen, depressive: this person pushed me away. When I was away researching this book, Seth had an affair. We went to therapy. He started spending nights away and, when he was home, downstairs on the couch. In therapy, he said he loved me but he just didn't know anymore. I tried to empathize, but really I was desperate: I raged, I sobbed, I clung in those long and terrible months. He stopped wearing his wedding ring, and then I claimed I couldn't read the signs. Empathy, I learned, is impossible when the life you know is threatened.

Or maybe we never really knew how to empathize with those closest to us, but rather only to mirror and to twin. When Seth broke that mirror, I was the one who shattered. One night he punched me in the face; I taught class the next day with a black eye, rode the subway in sunglasses. I didn't leave right away, but I knew that soon I would have to. If once I had cherished Seth more than my fears, had lived out a journey to help him be more alive, I would now have to flip the script and nourish my own life, and self, even more.

The trouble was, there wasn't much of a self to turn to, inextricably bound with Seth as it was. And I realized, as I was writing this book on empathy, that I was a fraud. I understood nothing about it at all.

When I began this project, I wore my smugness openly. I thought I was in an empathic relationship, thought I had read enough about empathy to understand it, and thought that when I turned up the volume on the current conversations on self-empathy happening all over the country, I would disparage them.

Until now, when I find myself alone in a one-bedroom apartment where I've moved to escape the pain of my relationship and the pain is all inside. There's no one here to empathize with me but me, and I don't know how to do it. This might be the hardest empathy of all.

. . .

IN A THERAPEUTIC SETTING, empathy is perceived as neither a skill nor a virtue but rather a complex interplay of an ability, an experience, a mode of communication, a form of data-gathering, a capacity, a process, an ego expression, a means of understanding, and a mode of perceiving. The psychologist Heinz Kohut is often credited with "inventing empathy" for the psychoanalytic field, but he really just put the emphasis there—radically transforming the therapeutic stance from one of a dispassionate observation to one of empathy. In the 1950s, Kohut broke with Freudian ideas around an individual's drives and the id, ego, and superego, and began to think primarily about an individual's relationships with others. To be overly simplistic, he thought that children developed their sense of self by both idealizing and emotionally sinking into people they admired, and by having their caregivers empathize with them and reflect back their own self-worth. In the 1970s, he formally introduced empathy right into the center of psychoanalytic theory and technique: if the therapist could adopt a primarily empathic stance, she could repair some of the failed or nonexistent empathy the patient experienced early on. One key to Kohutian theory is this: patients become patients because they've failed to develop self-empathy. When primary objects (parents, mainly) don't empathize with an infant's or child's failures and difficulties and respond appropriately, the child can't internalize that empathy and can't manage painful and difficult moments on his own. Clinicians can empathize and thereby teach it again.

But empathy in itself, Kohut stresses, is value-neutral. It can be employed in the service of compassion or hostility (think of the ways a sadist must understand his victim's fears). While empathy is a precondition for a parent's proper response to a child's suffering, it's only a first step. The next is to meet the child's needs—for comfort, for calming, whatever. When parents do this, they become for the child what Kohut calls a "selfobject"—people, objects, or activities that unconsciously but powerfully complete the self and are necessary for its functioning.

As a baby, I know, my selfobjects were inconsistent and some-times very frightening. My father was stable and loved me, and he said my mother was "good with babies," but by the time I have con-scious memories, she was already riding her psychotic swells. We lived in a suburb of San Francisco, which, my mother said, coolly dripped a poison into its inhabitants via the fog. She alternately told me that my birth had taken place in a hospital, in an army tent with scant supplies, and on the back of a camel. When I was eight, and my father had left, she gave me a deadbolt for my room to protect me from all the night men she said were clients, and perhaps from her as well. But she also was like a little girl, prone to pink sweat-ers and to crying all night when she misplaced one of her countless porcelain kittens. I can't imagine that this mom only appeared with the onset of memory, can't believe that she perfectly hinged onto my infant needs only to crack and crumble later. I can't imagine it because I left my mother's house when I was fourteen years old, and I never saw her again. And now, even with her eight years dead, I can't think of her without a kind of terror sawing through me. This terror is primal, preverbal, unyielding, and everything I know.

Kohut believed that we continue to incorporate selfobjects throughout our lives, though none are as primary as those initial caregivers. So I imagine Seth was a selfobject for me, a stabilizer and a promise—a sort of outer limit to my early and ongoing sense that I am forever falling. When he left, he razored a hole in the cap of that sanity. Kohut would say we internalize our selfobjects, so when the objects go, we still carry their imprint and their gifts. My thera-pist would say it's time for me to become the outer limits for myself, which is really the same thing. But I would say Seth took me with him; there was little me, without that us, to hold.

All of this is to say I don't know about self-empathy when the self is rendered fragmentary, dissolute. And I don't know about generating empathy in classrooms or courtrooms or country disputes when families are the seat of our sorrows, and so often, we can't find empathy there.

I thought a lot about this last idea even before Seth and I separated, felt it as a source of fraudulence within. If I couldn't generate empathy for my own family of origin, I wondered, how could I hope for more? My father and stepmother and I speak very rarely, so there's little chance for a direct empathic exchange; my brother and I do not speak at all. I think the root of this estrangement is my mother, or rather, the stories we tell about her. It's uncomfortable, and patently unfair, to speak for any of them on a page where they have no standing, but my father, I think it's safe to say, wishes I would tell the good parts, where he is loving and alert, a man who forged a new family in the wake of some pain best left forgotten. But that pain has shaped me for walking forward, and I've refused to lie still. When I speak, he changes the terms, believing we've come to some sort of agreement, and I die a little inside, determined to never speak to him in any real way again.

This dynamic makes me almost unbearably sad, though I think it is common enough. Children, once reliant on their parents to self-actualize, will use that self-actualization to reject their parents' ways. And perhaps that's what my father gave me — the strength to say a silent no. Still, I see his stance as a narcissistic one, though perhaps he sees mine that way too. I watch him become injured and enraged when another truth, mine for instance, encroaches upon his own. There isn't room for multiplicity — a space, I think, where empathy could take hold. His versions of my life and our shared history are absolute, inflexible, and so I step away, wondering if empathy from afar is empathy at all. Because I can generate kindness for the staunch father in my mind, but perhaps this is gestural, patronizing, designed only to mask the sting of one more loss.

Narcissism was a central theme for Kohut, though his optimistic view was largely misinterpreted amid the noisy cultural clamor in the 1970s lamenting the rise of an American narcissism that was poised as consumerist, shallow, and self-interested. The *New York Times* heralded an Age of Narcissism in the early 1970s, and Christopher Lasch's landmark 1979 book, *The Culture of Narcissism,* was a bestseller and a National Book Award winner. Borrowing heavily from Kohut's contemporary Otto Kernberg (who wrote about malignant narcissism), Lasch's thesis was that, after World War II, America had produced a unique personality type consistent with pathological narcissism, and we were in some deep trouble. Lasch cited everything from radical political activism to personal growth movements to support his claim, and the individual figure that emerged was superficial and sociable, unempathically self-serving but internally weak, with a low self-esteem, hungry for endless gratification and praise.

Kohut, bucking the trend around him, saw that the cultural emptiness and fragmentation resulted from not too much narcissism but too little. For him, narcissism was a healthy route to independence, satisfaction, and wholeness in the face of society's splintering demands. This particular idea wasn't woven into the larger dialogue about narcissism, but an attendant one was, particularly over time: Kohut thought that the way to treat narcissism, clinically, was with empathy. He advocated meeting narcissists' needs, and supporting their aspirations, however grandiose, empathically. This last notion seems to have stuck, since most of the literature suggests that narcissism, as a diagnosis, is hard to treat (for one, patients don't stay in treatment), and a nonconfrontational, empathic stance is the only fruitful approach.

Psychiatry historian Elizabeth Lunbeck argues in her book *The Americanization of Narcissism* that the narcissism name-calling craze of the 1970s was a ruse for a story each generation tells about the next: the youth have lost their values. They're out for themselves instead of for the common good. They've forgotten about the family. And yet it's a story we continue to tell. The Me Generation that

Lasch and other social critics lamented was followed by the lost and selfish Generation X, and now we have the navel-gazing, twittering Millennials (often dubbed Generation Me). So I wonder if this is the mantle we wear: in our collective call for treatment, we call for empathy.

At the Mindful Self-Compassion workshop, my resistance may have come from a traumatic past, as Chris Germer suggested, or from the outlook of a too-cramped calendar. But there was another path to self-compassion on offer that weekend, outside of Germer's head-on version.

Richard Schwartz was a co-presenter at the conference and the creator of a well-established psychological modality called Internal Family Systems (IFS). He began by telling us the story of the way he started IFS. It was born from his work with patients who had a hard time generating self-empathy.

The story went like this: it was the 1990s, and Schwartz was working with cutters and bingers. He said the patients who binged, for instance, claimed that when something bad happened in their lives, the binge rescued them, made them feel better. But the binge brought on the inner critic who was punitive and called them names, which brought on the purge — and thus the cycle would begin again. Like most in his field, Schwartz conceptualized the critical voice inside as an internalized parent — and he worked to get his patients to try to stand up to that voice, to control the binge. He did the same with the cutters.

With one particular client, Schwartz said, "I decided I wasn't going to let her leave my office until the part [the region of her psyche that wanted to self-harm] had agreed not to cut anymore. Two and a half hours later, with me badgering this part of her, it agreed not to do it. Of course, I opened the door the next session, and now she's got a big gash down the side of her face. I collapsed at that point and just said, 'I give up.' That was a historic moment because I shifted out of that more coercive part of me to just flat-out curiosity." At that point, Schwartz continued, he began to ask the cutting part questions. The cutting part told the story of how much she had been abused, and explained that the cutting helped her get out of her body, which helped her contain the rage, which brought on more abuse.

"I shifted again. Now I don't just have curiosity about it, but I have an appreciation for the heroic role it played in her life. I could extend that compassion to this part, and the part burst into tears because everyone had demonized and tried to get rid of it," he said. "The part talked more about how it still needed to protect other parts of her that were still very vulnerable and how it was stuck in her past and so on."

This was the basis of IFS. Schwartz went on to map a complex cosmology of parts and the way they operate and interact with one another, but the central theory is this: we all have multiple personalities, or parts, within us. It's the nature of the mind to be subdivided that way. Amid all these parts is a Self: a competent, secure, relaxed center. Ideally, this Self should be running the ship, but often one of the parts takes over and says, I'm a mean person, an insecure person, a weak person, whatever—and that's who we believe we *are*. The trick is to talk to these parts, ask them what they're doing, which exiled emotions they're covering. The trick is to move with compassion.

"You don't have to believe in the ontological reality of this, but most everybody can find these different parts and relate to them in a much more compassionate way," Schwartz said. When we do this, "the parts will actually start to transform."

I suddenly realized why I couldn't easily empathize with myself, as Germer proposed it, with MSC. That self I'd felt myself to be, through the long breakup with Seth, wasn't a self with a capital S at all. That self was a part—which felt fragmented, abandoned, terrified to be alone. And that part harkened back to a younger me, living with a mother who felt exactly the same way.

When practicing self-compassion, Schwartz told the group, "you need to ask, 'Who's being compassionate to whom?'" In other words, if a part is dominating the psyche and, like me, crying out in terror and desperation, that part can't very well exercise much kindness. It can't do much more than scream. To work with this, Schwartz will prompt a client to ask this dominant part to step back a little, and then to ask it questions. By doing this, he said, "their hearts would open. They would have compassion for this part instead of battling all the time and would reveal what it was protecting, what it was afraid would happen if it didn't constantly nag at the moment." In doing that, the dominant part would point toward the exiled feelings. "It would point toward these very vulnerable parts that it was so afraid would be triggered."

So I thought about it. I sat with Schwartz's concepts a long time. His process seemed intuitive, facile, productive. And I found that the part that says I am a terrified person is in fact covering and protecting an exiled feeling that I don't want to know.

When I was a very young child, I believe I was like most children: I wanted to be in the world. My first word was "wassat?" But I grew up with a psychotic mother; I grew up with someone who swirled me into her madness, and I attached deeply in that place. With my mother I was skinless; I tried to take care of her, but I also became her. Sometimes I felt as though we shared a circulatory system. And so to feel the world was to feel her loss — vast, empty, terrifying. She didn't live in the touchable, breathable world that I wanted to access; she lived with the demons of her mind, and so when I finally ran from her at fourteen, I couldn't be alone. To do that would be to betray the way she had taught me to commune, and to access my profound deprivation at once. I had to merge with someone, somewhere, to not feel the loss of never having lived.

I tried to merge with my father, and that worked for a while, until it didn't. My father and stepmother, with whom I lived in high school, wanted us all to be the same, to project an image of family that was charming, unified, unblemished by individuated needs. When I came out and they rejected me, I braided myself into the lives of lovers. From age twenty to thirty-six, I was married to one woman; from thirty-six until our breakup, I was with Seth, shouting that I couldn't be alone.

That day at the conference, seeing this fear as a part, rather than some kind of inherent, unhingeable me, did unleash some compassion. I was suddenly sad that I've spent most of my life prostrate to the straw god of fear inside, that I always did have more on offer. That fear was covering a feeling—one of open, gorgeous curiosity shot through with deep loss.

"As certain parts separate, immediately or spontaneously this other person shows up who knows how to relate to these parts in a healing way," Schwartz said. This other person is what he came to call the Self, but when this Self started appearing early on in his work, "I became very confused because I had been taught that for people to have that kind of ego strength inside, they needed to have had a certain kind of parenting at a certain critical period in their lives. Many of my clients had been tortured on a daily basis, and there was no way to account for all this strength."

Because Schwartz couldn't ground this observation in psychoanalytic doctrine, he had to shift toward spiritual writings. "Scriptural traditions have a word for this experience and know about it—in Buddhism, it's called Buddha-nature—but very few psychotherapists do."

In my family—when we do communicate—none of us are operating from this Self. I haven't seen my father and stepmother for seven years, and even then just for a coffee. With my brother, it's been longer. Aside from generating an extravagant guilt hemmed in by outsize fear, this separation has fueled my sense of imposture as I've explored the larger project of empathy. Again, I've thought, if I (and likely others) can't muster empathy for the roots that grew me, how legitimate are the empathetic fruits I bear for others?

But it's easier to find this generous Self when I'm with other people, when my parts, as Schwartz would call them, aren't directing the show. When I'm with my family, I narrow down to memory, eclipsing potential for broader vision, and I suspect my family members do the same. I am simply seven or ten or fifteen years old again, still breathing my mother's air and terrified of being consumed.

Very recently, my father and stepmother and I have been trying to set up a get-together: we would all like to reconcile in some way. But we can't agree to the terms. I would like a mediator, but they don't welcome a third party, so I'm not sure we'll even make it to the front door. I would like to find a way to understand our divergent experiences and pains, to listen to one another, perhaps, to empathize. They've said they want to drop the old pains and move on. I'm not sure I can cosign their goal.

So perhaps my ambition is unrealistic. And maybe, I suspect, my real goal — simply because the relationship is so deep and so old — is not just to empathize but to forgive.

Conventional theories of forgiveness involve an expression of remorse. Some have written that, in the face of violations, remorse is a vital ingredient for empathy too. I know, however, I won't get that; no apology will tumble from my parents' mouths, especially as they want to drop old pains and move on. I know too that this is a child's wish, a fantasy that a single sorry can make history wash away.

And in reality, I'm too steeped in my years of therapy to really believe in this curative potential. (Psychoanalysis as a field has held a contentious relationship with forgiveness, ever since Freud — who maintained that forgiveness wasn't possible in a human unconscious so riddled with ambivalence.) So why do I want it? Professor and political psychologist C. Fred Alford suggests that the wish to forgive is a wish to preserve the familiar people we all were back when original wounds were inflicted. But of course this is impossible. Instead, we have to mourn the ways those people are gone.

Judith Butler, in her book *Precarious Life: The Powers of Mourning and Violence,* writes about the transformational — and frightening — potential of this mourning. She observes, "On one level, I think I have lost 'you' only to discover that 'I' have gone missing as well."

Given that I feel so young and stuck when I am with my family, this interpretation makes a lot of sense to me. Alford takes it further, though, and says that, ironically, when we do mourn the old self or part and thereby let it go, we enter a space where forgiveness, or empathy, becomes possible — spontaneously, in its own time, and not necessarily through any kind of direct or spoken interchange. This idea parallels Schwartz's work with parts: when one difficult, controlling part can soften or step aside, a more generous, forgiving, empathizing Self will step in.

In that vein, I recently asked my father, on his seventieth birthday, if he'd like to start exchanging letters — gentle ones, not about anything particular or charged, just gestures of connection without the burden of expectation. He agreed, and we've sent a few back and forth. He started by telling me who he is now — what he does with his time, whom he loves spending it with, and so forth. I told him what I'm currently reading. Our words are all in present tense; we don't touch upon the pasts, which are separate and ours to mitigate alone. The letters are careful and mannered and lovely in their way, and maybe, I think, something new can be born there.

9

State of Empathy

The airport in Bangor, Maine, is the entry to the third-largest city in the state and the picture of small-town America. The single terminal hosts a sandwich shop, a bank of old pay phones, and several glass display cases showcasing the wares of the stores on Main Street. When I went to Bangor in the spring of 2015, I was deep in my breakup with Seth and so wondering about the ways personal heartbreak extends to the workings of trauma across generations, about whether forgiveness on an individual level can help heal violations deeper or larger than a single person can commit. In no way was I trying to equate my personal history with larger-state violations but I was thinking about empathy's curative potential, on both a large and small stage, and Maine had just completed a project to look at just that.

The glass cases in the airport were paeans to patriotism: one featured red-and-white tulips atop a starry blue cloth; a jewelry store flew an enormous crystal bald eagle in front of the American flag. But beneath all this kitschy, boisterous pride is another, very American story. This story is old and layered and full of cruelty and heartbreak — so people don't like to tell it much. Maine's story of Native American genocide and subsequent centuries of abuse and resilience is similar to other states', but in the past few years, Maine has embarked on a vigorous project to look at it, to talk about it, and to understand. With all five tribes and representatives from the state of Maine, they've just completed a new kind of Truth and Reconciliation Commission (TRC), and it's an empathic example unlike any other. Fostering empathy for the enemy is difficult, especially when that enemy tracks back hundreds of years and is a faceless state, but the TRC was not just about providing a forum for empathic listening. It offered a context that unveiled historical complexity and culpability and the multigenerational traumas which linked the murders of the past to the loss and confusion of right now. The TRC also established platforms for future healing, so in this way it spans past, present, and future, and has more potential as a comprehensive model for executing broad-based empathy in this country than any other I've seen.

All over the world, there are hot spots where one group of people has committed gross human rights violations against another and then, in an attempt to heal or perhaps to simply live alongside one another again, these groups have to forge some sort of forgiveness. They have to broker an understanding. In studying the Maine Wabanaki TRC, I've found that this last and largest form of empathy isn't really so different from the other forms I've explored in that, while the end results may be grander, its roots are usually about one-to-one exchanges. One human being empathizes, and perhaps forgives, another human being, and in that interchange imaginatively extends goodwill to the broader state.

The TRC began humbly in an office in 1999 when some state workers sat down with tribal representatives to talk about the gaps and failures in the state-run foster care system. Nationally, child welfare is one of the particularly shameful areas of state-sponsored abuse in Native communities: in the late 1800s, Native children were forcibly removed from their homes and institutionalized in boarding schools, a practice that continued into the early twentieth century. Boarding schools were replaced in the 1950s by the federally financed Indian Adoption Project. Somewhere between 25 and 35 percent of all Indian children were removed from their homes and placed with white families. By 1978, on paper at least, this had turned around, with the Indian Child Welfare Act (ICWA), which seeks to keep Indian kids with Indian families. But by then, in Maine, too many kids were already gone: Maine had the second-highest rate of Indian foster care placement in the country.

And despite ICWA, the culture was set: throughout the 1990s, child welfare workers continued to remove Native kids from their families and place them with and adopt them into white families. At the time of the 1999 meeting, one of the Maine tribes still had 16 percent of its kids in state custody—in direct opposition to ICWA mandates. The idea then was to create a workgroup to better comply with ICWA and rewrite policy, and to start a dialogue between tribal and state child welfare agencies.

That dialogue, however, was fraught and untrusting right from the beginning. Penthea Burns was a caseworker for the state in 1999 and attended that meeting. "The tribal people had no faith in the state government entering into this in a genuine kind of way because of everything they had experienced. The folks from the different tribes had not sat in a room together, so they didn't have any reason to trust one another. The tension was honestly—well, I felt like I could see ghosts in the room," she said. Burns is a white woman in her fifties, with short grey hair and deep brown eyes. She's a poet and has a grounded, calming air about her. On winter weekends, she goes sledding with her dogs. "It didn't take long to realize, 'Oh, wait a minute, we really need the whole of tribal communities involved and we really need the whole of Maine involved.'"

That's because nobody could contain the problem to 1999; nobody could discuss the solutions to ICWA without exposing the violations that came before. In fact, the issues were so enormous, it took thirteen more years of meetings to shape, develop, and launch what would eventually become the Maine Wabanaki Child Welfare Truth and Reconciliation Commission. Part of the reason for the pace was fear. Esther Attean, a member of the Passamaquoddy tribe and now co-director of Maine-Wabanaki REACH, which provides support and resources for the TRC, was at that initial meeting too, and deeply involved in all the subsequent planning. Esther is lean and darting, with a piercing look and a fast, brassy laugh. She folds herself into chairs rather than sits in them, and though she's a grandmother, she springs up with the energy of a teenager. "I remember one day just the anxiety and the fear was so high. Somebody said, 'We can't do this, this is wrong, because as soon as people start talking about this, people are going to start drinking and drugging and killing themselves,'" she said. "And then we stopped and said, 'You know what? We're already doing that. The silence is not working for us.'"

In June 2012, leaders of the five Wabanaki tribal governments sat beside the Republican governor, Paul LePage, to sign the mandate of Maine's first TRC. At a basic level, the idea was to gather statements from all indigenous and nonindigenous people who had been involved with child welfare since 1978, the year ICWA passed. In reality, the TRC would look all the way back into the sixteenth century and forward deep into the twenty-first century and involve the entire state of Maine.

In a project that spanned two years, the TRC gathered statements from 156 tribal members and people formerly involved with child welfare. The archive would be permanently housed and preserved at Bowdoin College. But more than that, they came up with action steps to reinforce healing and ongoing communication between the two formerly estranged groups. In studying this process, I learned that forging empathy between people and a faceless state that has committed grievous harm against them requires a grounding in deep education, new styles of listening, and sometimes no direct communication at all.

The most well-known truth and reconciliation commission was created in South Africa after apartheid. Rather than conduct

Nuremberg-style trials — the retributive justice approach to gross human rights violations by the state — Nelson Mandela and other leaders developed the TRC as a restorative option and a way to transition to full democracy. Both victims and perpetrators gave statements in courtrooms across the country, and some perpetrators were granted amnesty in exchange for their testimony. Dozens of TRCs have been established internationally since South Africa, in various styles and to varied success.

In Maine, Penthea Burns says they never considered facing the victims and perpetrators against one another, courtroom-style, the way they did in South Africa. "We never conceptualized it in that way, because we knew that the problems were about racism and privilege and power," she said. "It was more of a systemic issue."

So how do you get white people to talk about their individual culpability and experience removing children from Native families, and how do you get Native families to share their pain and rage and guilt over having their children taken, if the process is all cloaked in the collective name of "racism and power"?

The answer is you start with education. "We don't know the history better than anybody else," Esther Attean said to me. For both the tribal members and the (primarily white) people involved with child welfare, the TRC and REACH showed films and held talks before people gave their statements, so they would have some historical context for their actions in the 1980s and 1990s. This history dates back to the early sixteenth century, when Spain adopted the Requerimiento, which asserted that God, through Saint Peter and his historical successors, ruled the earth. This assertion granted the pope the authority to grant the title of all the Americas to the Spanish monarchs. These monarchs required that a doctrine of discovery be read (in Latin and Spanish) to all indigenous people upon encounter. Even though they couldn't understand the language, they were told, "If you do not do this [accept Spanish rule] and maliciously make delay in it, I certify to you, with the help of God, we shall powerfully enter your country, and shall make war against you . . . We shall take you, and your wives, and your children, and shall make slaves of them, and as such shall sell and dispose of them as their highnesses may command."

While the doctrine was ultimately abolished, the dogma persisted as colonizers changed shape. A man named Spencer Phips was governor of Massachusetts in 1755 (Maine was not yet a state) and issued a Bounty Proclamation offering fifty pounds for every Penobscot male (one of the Wabanaki tribes), forty pounds for just the scalp, and twenty pounds for the scalp of a woman or child. In the end, the Wabanaki lost 90 percent of their population in the genocide.

This education wends its way through the Indian boarding schools and the Indian Adoption Project, up to today when, despite ICWA, Maine's Native kids are still five times more likely than non-Native kids to be removed. Attean described this all as intergenerational trauma, which is "usually a combination of immense losses and takings, traumatic assaults, extreme hopelessness that's perpetuated upon an entire culture. It's cumulative and collective and it results in increasing emotional and physical, psychological wounding across generations." She likened the experience of being educated in this history to finally getting a diagnosis. She described the high levels of joblessness, dropout rates, and alcoholism. "It's easy to think that there's something wrong with you but there's nothing wrong with us at all; this is just how a population would look after hundreds of years of continued strategies and policies of genocide."

Attean said this educational foreground helped people with their guilt during the TRC statement-gathering, particularly for people whose children had been taken. "I remember this one guy, he was saying, 'I never can get anything right. I can't keep the job, I couldn't keep my kids.' That historical context really took a lot of blame from him," she said. "It created empathy for himself."

Aside from the education component, the TRC established different parameters for statement-gathering among the Wabanaki and former child welfare workers. The white respondents were asked a specific set of questions, whereas the Native respondents were encouraged to speak extemporaneously, beginning and ending in whatever portion of their story they felt comfortable. This was an attempt to circumvent retraumatization, as well as to honor a form of talking and listening that has always been foregrounded in Wabanaki communities.

I spoke a bit with one of the four TRC commissioners, a man named gkisedtanamoogk, about this listening. Gkisedtanamoogk teaches Native American studies at the University of Maine, has a mohawk and deep dimples, and several face tattoos. "In my culture we recognize that it's one thing to listen, it's another thing to hear, and most of the time we're hearing, we're not listening," he said. "Hearing means that you're just thinking about what you're going to say, you're thinking about your own thoughts, you're thinking about what's going to happen down the road. Listening means you put all that aside and you only focus on what's being said, you're not thinking about anything. Our purpose is to listen and to record. It's really important that the statement provider is not distracted by questions or anything of that nature: just listen."

Gkisedtanamoogk is Wampanoag, and he says, growing up, his tribe always held councils, which were open meetings. He described an environment where one or two people would discuss whatever issue was at hand, then pass around a council stick for people to reflect. There were no questions, no back-talk, no interruptions: as long as someone had the stick, she could talk forever. I raised my eyebrows and gkisedtanamoogk nodded. "Maybe there's a little bit of discipline for those who are not accustomed to that. There's a difference between interviewing state DHHS [Department of Health and Human Services] workers and tribal members. Tribal members will just share their story in narrative."

Esther Attean grew up at the Pleasant Point Reservation, where she says her mother remembers living without electricity (14 percent of Native households in the United States still don't have access to electricity). "Everybody would just sit around at night. People would talk, so we had that uninterrupted time," Attean recalled. She said her mother started a more formal group for women only, called the Screaming Eagles, where the idea was to listen to one another without thinking of anything but the person's unconditional goodness. It made some of the people in the community "really good listeners, with a really caring, conditional regard. You feel that love from them no matter what."

As Attean spoke, I wondered whether I had ever listened in quite that way before, with the attention on someone's goodness or humanity. I certainly wasn't doing it then, wasn't focusing solely on Attean's words or affect or meaning, without looping back to self-scan. After all, the most salient definitions of empathy delineate some kind of self-other kickback, and I was practicing what I'd been preached. Unlike the class I'd taken on empathic listening where I'd learned to interrogate the other and then interrogate myself, searching for wants and needs, which had felt entirely immediate and intuitive, this one-way channel would take work.

I met with Attean at the Wabanaki Health and Wellness Center, a two-story building in downtown Bangor that provides services like housing referrals and case management. We were joined by Sharon Tomah, the director, who recruited Wabanaki people to give statements to the TRC and shares gkisedtanamoogk's and Attean's philosophy that listening empathically is primarily a generous and unreflective process. "I believe that empathy is a capacity to really understand and feel what the experience of someone else is and to give of yourself generously in all different ways—spiritually, cognitively, physically, or whatever," Tomah said.

To provide the widest opportunity for this kind of empathic listening, the TRC did more than just one-on-one statement-gathering on the Wabanaki side. For people who wanted a roomful of support, they held healing circles where anyone could speak without a recorder. These circles were private, so I couldn't attend, but Attean said sometimes these would warm people up a bit, and they'd decide to then tell their story on record. Sometimes, however, people would attend the circles and opt out from the statements entirely.

"One particular family was doing the circles, they had been in horrendous foster homes and just so grossly mistreated and abused and bullied. One of the brothers was so angry about it, and I was really hoping he would give a statement and he said, 'Yep, I'm going to be there. I'm going to be there,'" Attean recalled. "At the last minute, he said, 'No, I can't do it, I just can't go there again. I can't let myself feel that again.'"

Both Attean and Tomah gave statements to the commission, and both had mixed feelings. Because their words would be saved in perpetuity, they were worried about hurting family members. "My aunt and stuff are still alive, and I have an understanding of why they couldn't take care of their kids and all that," Attean said, rushing her words even more than usual. "But there was that worry about publicly shaming them in the community."

Tomah, at first, didn't want to give her statement at all. "I could have easily not have done it," she said, explaining that her great-niece was removed from the family and put into foster care. As the director of Wabanaki Wellness and a therapist there, Tomah sees lots of families hurt by chronic lack of opportunity and its subsequent depression — which, she says, can manifest like mental illness and be the ostensible cause for a child's removal. In my own work in foster care, I know the frustration of this cycle: children are removed from families because the parents are behaving in an acutely dangerous way. The root of the problem, however, lies elsewhere — to use a kind of shorthand, in poverty and discrimination. Addressing that larger problem by removing a child is like fixing the flu with some lip balm—except in this case, the balm becomes a trauma for everyone involved. "In the end, I said to hell with it, I'll tell the story. It just wasn't as easy as I thought it was going to be, going there again."

All told, after two full years of statement-gathering, ninety-two Wabanaki people gave official signed statements to the TRC and many more told their stories in healing circles. Generally, TRC members would come into a town or community and spend a whole day: holding circles and showing films, gathering statements and reflecting, praying and meditating at the end. While the official TRC work is done, REACH, the support organization, will continue. One of the prime goals for the TRC, aside from documenting a mostly silent history, was to discern from the testimony the tangible actions that might prevent child welfare atrocities again.

To a packed auditorium in Bangor, the commissioners presented these steps. It was the first of four major presentations to be held in cities across the state to share the mandate and results of the two-year TRC process. Several audience members came carrying trays of homemade brownies or finger sandwiches or reused milk jugs bearing iced tea for everyone to share after the meeting. A large sheet cake read "Beyond the Mandate" in scripted frosting. "It feels important to recognize that we are in the Dyke Center at Husson College in Bangor, Maine, on Penobscot territory, and to be very aware of all that's come before in this spot," the elder commissioner Carol Wishcamper said by way of opening. It didn't look like we were on Penobscot territory. The college has a neatly manicured, suburban golf-course-cum-office-park feel. It's perched on a slight hill surrounded by a neighborhood of two-story clapboard homes. Of course, all of Maine was Wabanaki territory at one time, and all of the presenters pressed on the notion that history is embedded in contemporary losses.

The first, and most basic, recommendation was to respect tribal sovereignty—to see Indian nations' laws and customs as distinct from the nation that contains them. Rigorously adapting this mind-set could help child welfare workers pause before they utilized their own mandates to remove children from difficult homes.

"Respect" is an interesting word when it comes to empathy. For those of us in the so-called helping positions, like social work, we may be told to empathize with our clients, but we're often caught in a dichotomy that makes real empathy impossible. The dichotomy is between agency and victimhood. The targets of social welfare programs are sometimes posited as victims—of institutionalized racism, generational poverty, and so forth. (The sex workers, for instance, who are brought before the human trafficking courts are positioned as these types of victims.) These victims are deserving of help. Or else they're agents—drug users, child neglecters, job avoiders, and so on. These agents don't deserve help. Rarely can they be both: in fact, the very idea of giving agents help, we say, is to treat them as victims, as though a person flips neatly between one and the other.

The answer might be to offer dignity first, which is a kind of respect. Philosopher Martha Nussbaum sees a finely wrought relationship between victimhood and agency. She says that injustice "can strike its roots into the personality itself, producing rage and resentment and the roots of bad character." She claims the way through the dichotomy is dignity: recognizing another human's basic dignity means seeing his agency within his victimization. Recognizing, and continually reifying, tribal sovereignty seem to me to be this kind of dignity.

The TRC's second recommendation was to honor and build tribal culture and traditions. This will bolster the community so that families within, perhaps, struggle just a bit less. Both Esther Attean and gkisedtanamoogk talked to me about the cultural renaissance newly flourishing in the tribes, especially in the ways young people were learning and speaking the languages, but REACH is developing programming for more ongoing traditional experiences

in all five reservation areas. One of the critiques of many TRCs is
that when they're over, people can't see the lasting effects, so Attean
said they'll be working with the tribes for many years to incorporate
birth, death, and coming-of-age rituals, as well as trainings in food
and medicine. She said, "If we can decolonize how we come into and
leave the world, those are two pretty strong actions of sovereignty."

The third recommendation was for white people, and REACH
will be facilitating that as well. Charlotte Bacon, the executive director of the TRC, took the mic. "This is easy to say and harder to do.
We need to develop trainings that really push people to look at their
privilege, to look at where they come from, to engage in self-reflec-
tion," she said, "so that every person who intersects with the child
welfare system in this state has done very deep inventories about
who they are, what they stand for, what they carry that is incredibly
positive and what they carry that they want to lay down."

REACH had already been doing these trainings when I went
to Maine, a series of workshops for allies to learn about Wabanaki
history and their own internalized racism and colonialism. Several
people told me the sessions had been well attended thus far. People tended to come away inspired to take action, but Penthea Burns
encourages people to slow down. "For those who are new to the
history, you want to fix stuff now, you want to make things better
now," she said. "But truly our job as allies is not to get in the middle
of Wabanaki communities but to get in the middle of ourselves and
ask, 'How do I reconcile who I thought I was with who I am now
that I know what happened in this state and in this country?'"

This impulse to fix is an impulse that planners were trying to
forestall in the early drafting of the TRC. "Often in truth and reconciliation processes, the group of people who have been oppressed
wants the truth to come out," Burns said. "The people who have
been a part of the group that was the oppressor wants to get to reconciliation."

This is part of the reason that, in statement-gathering, questions for state workers were more guided. The point wasn't ever to assign blame but rather to first introduce the history so the workers, like the Wabanaki participants, could see they were part of a larger system. Then they'd be asked technical questions about types of removals in particular geographic locations as well as what they felt good about in their work with Native kids and what, perhaps, they wished had been different. In all, sixty-four caseworkers, supervisors, administrators, attorneys, as well as foster and adoptive parents, gave statements to the commission.

A woman named Barbara Kates was in charge of coordinating many of the interviews with the state workers. I met with her at her home. We ate cherry apple pie and sipped tea in Kates's peacock-blue living room filled with spider plants and tapestries as she told me that about half the people she reached out to wouldn't talk to the commission at all.

"They were concerned about their information being taken out of context," she explained. "They felt like they've worked really hard to have positive relationships with Wabanaki people, and they were afraid if they'd be put in a position to share their misgivings, it would hurt their current relationships."

Penthea Burns gave a testimony to the commission, and it wasn't what she remembered about her time as a child welfare worker that was painful — but what she didn't. "It had been a long time since I thought back to being a caseworker," she said, explaining that in general, she was so caught up in the flow of cases, she didn't stop to ask whether someone was a Native child or fell under ICWA jurisdiction. "It wasn't even avoidance," she said sadly. "It was like beneath that. I didn't exercise any curiosity to do anything more."

I've studied foster care for years and have found that malice and ill-intent are rare: it's an overburdened system pulled at all sides by conflicting interests. Caseworkers are at the center of this storm, very often relegated to the short view that emergencies require. So I understand why workers would be reluctant to pause and reflect for the TRC: they were afraid, after serving only one cog, that they'd suddenly have to take responsibility for the whole machine.

Still, Kates said, that largely didn't happen: "You could see, when people walked in to give their statements, their shoulders were up, you could feel the tension. When they walked out, their shoulders were down, and most people would tell me they were glad they came." Many people felt as if they didn't have a story to tell at all. Like Burns, they just remembered a generalized lack of attention to Native kids—which led to all the excess placements in white homes. But with a little probing, things would come back. In her testimony, Burns remembered a Native boy who was from a tribe outside of Maine. She passed the case on to her supervisor and didn't follow up.

Part of the TRC's mandate was to take statements like Burns's and cross-reference them with the state archives to track cases and develop a full and accurate accounting of all the Native transfers into white households since 1978. This is the technical seam they're stitching between the Wabanaki tribes and the state; the emotional one is harder. In many TRCs, the two sides of a conflict will present their statements to one another, in a twinned act of confrontation and healing. In Maine, however, the state and tribal components operated independently, and statements were given in private—only to commingle later, as one large document, and to be paraded out at public gatherings.

I've thought a lot about the efficacy of the Maine approach in terms of building empathy between distrustful sets of people. On one hand, it's safer—as a platform for the initial telling, keeping stories in-group can evoke more candid expression, without fear of immediate repercussion. This recorded, "truer" story can then be shared in mixed company. On the other, the victim in this version doesn't ever get to face her perpetrator head-on. This, to me, seems one direct and immediate form of reconciliation. And, perhaps, another stage of empathy.

This last idea, granted, was never an objective for the Maine-

Wabanaki TRC. In their initial mandate, their goals were to "give voice to the Wabanaki people with experience in child welfare," and to all those who worked with Wabanaki families from 1978 until today. From this, they wanted to create "opportunities for healing" and a "deeper understanding" between the two groups. They looked to build a more complete history of what happened in those years and formulate better standards and practices for a system going forward. Finally—and these are the big ones—they wanted to come up with recommendations so that the "lessons of truth are not forgotten" and to "promote individual, relational, systemic and cultural reconciliation."

Our collective human psyche grips tightly to the promise of "never forget" whenever the state commits gross human rights abuses, whenever it's safe again to make that promise. One of the early truth commissions, after the dirty war in Argentina, was called Nunca Mas, and that prophylactic function is implicit in the never forgetting: we remember so as not to repeat.

But "truth" is a small word to shoulder so many demands, and shared facts don't always cohere into shared truths. In many oppressive regimes, the oppressors' truth is that they were following orders, believing they were fighting an enemy. In South Africa, security forces believed they were protecting the country from communist insurgents; in Maine, they were protecting innocent children.

Getting from these divergent truths to reconciliation usually involves acknowledgment and contrition from the perpetrators—a form of remorse—and then forgiveness for the perpetrators. But this means, first, seeing the others' truth and understanding it. And for this, there has to be a platform. In South Africa, the platform was generally a courtroom or other public space where victims and perpetrators were confined to the same area and compelled to listen to the others' testimony. Very often spontaneous acts of remorse, forgiveness, and reconciliation were enacted upon those stages. Because these acts were televised, the idea was to elevate the personal reconciliation to the national, as individual bodies stood in for larger atrocities.

Critics of the TRC said perpetrators were paying for their freedom with truth. Offering amnesty for a full narrative account of one's crimes wasn't truth at all, some said: it was a free pass. And yet, in Maine, where the potentially criminal acts weren't personal but rather framed as historic and systemic, where no one was forced to appear before tribunals, and where amnesty was neither proffered nor given, only half of the state workers chose to meet with the commission. So they probably weren't getting a full picture there either.

Still, Sharon Tomah told me she was surprised that so many state workers and non-Native people volunteered to come forth. "I had a hard time believing people would care, since they weren't mandated to be involved, but this whole project has taught me something different," she said, citing not only the people who provided formal statements but also those who continue to attend the ally workshops and public forums. "Maybe that's because I haven't seen evidence of it before and because of that internalized depression which says we really aren't important, we really don't matter to anybody."

It's at the forums that commissioners will air some of the taped testimony. I witnessed one such story. In the auditorium at Husson University, they darkened the room and lowered a screen. An older woman, rubbing her hands together, spoke on film.

"I can't get over the nightmares. All we did was beg for our foster mother to hug us and say they loved us. My baby sister and I sat in a tub of bleach one time, tried to convince each other that we're getting white, and then we knew they would accept us," she said. "Where was the state? Where was the state that was supposed to have been our guardians? Where were they? They weren't there for us. We knew nothing else but foster people. How come it took so long for you all to get a group together to see if they can help us? You can't heal someone that's gone through hell."

And yet these private disclosures, made public, do a sort of healing work. After the film, Esther Attean said, a young man came up to her, wanting to talk. He hadn't been involved in any statement-gathering or healing circles; he preferred the anonymity of the larger community presentation. In one of the clips we watched, he saw his grandmother's sister. "And he goes, 'Oh my God, I didn't realize.' A lightbulb went off," she said, explaining that this person had been in jail and separated from his kids. He'd only focused on that singular aspect of his experience, and connecting it to a longer string of history "created empathy and understanding for his parents, his grandparents and for himself."

At another one of the presentations, Penthea Burns said, a former caseworker stood up at the very end of the question-and-answer period to make a public confession. "This little bitty woman stands up in the back of the room, and she said, 'I'm here. I used to be a caseworker with the state. I took your children and I'm here to say I'm sorry.' You could hear a pin drop in the room," Burns said. These kinds of spontaneous acts of contrition can be reconciliatory, but for this particular TRC, the goal was to build empathy and understanding between the groups, not necessarily make the leap to forgiveness. Attean responded to the woman and, Burns recalled, thanked her for speaking up. "She held that balance between graciousness but not overly caretaking or not giving her forgiveness. What Esther said is, 'I didn't feel like it was mine to give.'"

But then a more intimate, personal exchange transpired. A woman named Denise Altvater, a Passamaquoddy citizen who had spent some of her own childhood in foster care, made a beeline to the former state worker. Burns watched as "they took each other's hands and they just stood there with their foreheads leaning up against one another. A minute, a minute and a half might have passed," Burns remembered. "They never said a word and just stood there sort of holding each other. Then Denise kissed her on the forehead and stood back. They smiled at one another, and the woman turned and walked away."

In this way, empathy is a starting point for something more. Empathy creates a space, an opening, for spontaneous, unchoreographed connection; it's a way of listening that fosters the potential for deeper meaning—like forgiveness—down the line. One of the primary goals in the initial TRC mandate was to initiate better long-term communication between the state and the tribes that extended beyond child welfare and into all areas of tribal relations. When Governor LePage sat down with all five Wabanaki chiefs to sign the TRC agreement, it was a historic moment, given the centuries of abuse and mistrust. The photo shows the governor seated at the center of a long table, his round face content and proud above a tightly buttoned shirt and tie. That day he said he believed that his relations with the tribes had always been good but he wanted to repair the damage from prior administrations. But the week the TRC released their report, two years after the signing, everyone I met was talking about LePage and the first TRC recommendation: tribal sovereignty.

That very week, LePage had rescinded his own 2011 executive order that recognized the "special relationship" between the Wabanaki tribes and the state of Maine. That order had created a consultation policy for tribal input before laws affecting them were passed. On a Saturday, in an email, he revoked that order, claiming that his efforts to promote collaboration and communication were "unproductive because the State of Maine's interests were not respected in the ongoing relationship between sovereigns."

But which interests were those? After all, the TRC had been working steadily to create the most comprehensive collaboration between the state and tribes that Maine had ever known. From what I could see, goodwill and empathy were fine, as long as they didn't touch the money. While the TRC had been gathering statements about child welfare abuses, LePage had been trying to secure waterways on tribal lands for the state's energy use. The tribes wanted to keep their rivers for fishing, as they always had. I don't know, of course, whether the release of the TRC report had anything to do with LePage's actions, but when the tribes didn't budge, LePage revoked their sovereignty.

Chief Kirk Francis of the Penobscot nation was the first to issue a statement, saying that such a rescinding does "nothing but fuel an already volatile relationship." Penthea Burns admitted that she didn't feel much personal compassion for the governor, but given all of her time working with the TRC, she did find herself wanting to communicate in a different kind of way. She wished the two sides could just sit together and talk longer. "If that governor could simply have the capacity to just stay at the table and say, 'No, I disagree, let's talk some more,' that would be a monumental shift."

But while videotaped statements and history lessons and healing circles and mixed-group forums may lead, in a trickle-down way, to individual acts of forgiveness and reconciliation, they may not flow back upward toward the seats of power. LePage never shifted on his new executive order, and a few weeks later, three of the four tribes withdrew their representatives from the legislature entirely.

10

To Interrupt Power

After witnessing the truth and reconciliation process unfold in Maine, I was curious to go to the TRC birthplace, a place where state-sponsored genocide and state-sponsored empathy had erupted within the same decades. I wanted to go to one of the most difficult places on the planet—where communication, trust, and life itself had been seemingly irredeemably ruptured, a place where one man tried to change it all through a deep process of bearing witness to, and understanding, the other. I booked a ticket to South Africa.

My starting point, and main contact, was Dr. Pumla Gobodo-Madikizela, an original TRC member and the psychologist who wrote *A Human Being Died That Night,* about trying to forgive Eugene de Kock, the leader of apartheid's death squads. Gobodo-Madikizela was running an institute for trauma, reconciliation, and forgiveness at a former Afrikaans university in Bloemfontein, an Afrikaans stronghold. If there was ever a place to practice empathy, this was it.

Bloemfontein is a city of 250,000 in a landlocked state in the low grasslands center of the country. *Bloemfontein* literally translates to flower fountain, and there are rosebushes planted everywhere— in the city parks, in yards, in the little plots outside people's high fences and electric gates. This might be the first thing an American newcomer would notice upon landing in Bloemfontein or any other

South African city: all the houses are blockaded by an impressive, looming architecture of walls, looped on top with electrified barbed wire and signs that say "danger" in English, Afrikaans, and Zulu. That, and the fact there are no sidewalks. People walk right down the middle of the streets.

Traffic moves slowly in Bloem; it feels suburban with its stately, hidden houses, despite the fact that it's the judicial capital of the country. "Nothing really happens in Bloem," locals told me again and again—primary entertainments were the malls and local soccer games—and they urged me to see the more exciting Johannesburg or gorgeous Cape Town.

But I was interested in Bloemfontein because I had a chance to study something very small in an attempt to grasp something very large. The city is home to the University of the Free State (UFS), which had been an all-white Afrikaans school that integrated after democracy. A few years ago, some Afrikaner students there posted a racist video that went viral internationally, which prompted the university and then the national government to take swift action designed to build empathy and understanding between black and white students. It was unlike anything I'd ever seen in the United States, where most cases of discrimination are handled punitively. But, as one UFS student told me, "empathy is an interruption of power." This was a model of empathy I wanted to understand.

I also wanted to understand, through the close microcosm of the university, the South African notion of *ubuntu*—a sometimes contested but still pervasive humanistic form of empathy that infused politics and social relations. Ubuntu is understood as the essence of being human, and it means "interconnected" or "I am what I am because of who we all are." Ubuntu, as both a philosophy and a source of law, was a cornerstone of Nelson Mandela's new democracy (in the constitution it reads, "There is a need for understanding but not for vengeance, a need for reparation but not for retaliation, a need for *ubuntu* but not for victimization"), and it was indelibly woven into the moves the university made after the racist attack. If I could understand ubuntu in some smaller ways, I could move on to understand the greater human project in South Africa of engendering empathy for the enemy.

I checked in at a small guesthouse near the university, outfitted tastefully in dark wood and creamy whites with the requisite roses trailing about outdoors. The owner, a vivacious Afrikaans woman in her late sixties named Charlotte, offered to drive me to the campus, where I was to have a temporary office in Gobodo-Madikizela's institute. Charlotte's husband taught at the university, and she knew the place well.

"See? It's almost all black now," Charlotte said, waving her arm out the open car window as we drove slowly along the curved roads of the campus. But I didn't see what she saw. Students were everywhere, carrying books, clustered in groups, studying under trees in the bucolic spring weather. They were segregated—white girls leaned into white boys, black girls pressed together in line at a café —but it wasn't all black. A quarter of the students seemed to be white.

I later learned that the thirty-thousand-strong student body was split 70/30—a major change from when Charlotte moved to the city to raise her children in 1982. Back then, all classes were taught in Afrikaans; now the buildings are labeled "Physics" and "Fisika," and all professors must teach a double load in English and Afrikaans. Back when Charlotte was raising her children, blacks were forced to live in townships outside the city—something she discussed freely and with shocking racism.

"This used to be quite a normal neighborhood; blacks were given their own land," Charlotte said, waving again at some vague distance. "But they didn't take care of it."

When I protested that the creation of *bantu stans,* or segregated black "homelands," when all blacks were forced to carry passbooks inside their own country, was one of the core evils of apartheid,

Charlotte brushed me off as an ignorant outsider. "Many of them were given quite large gardens," she replied.

I felt sick, and I quickly realized that my first task, before I settled into the university to learn about its policies of empathic inclusion, would be to move. But then I discovered that finding someplace without traces of long-held racism would be difficult. This was a city that birthed the National Party, the party of apartheid, and where home ownership, and certainly guest lodgings, were disproportionately Afrikaner.

Attitudes like Charlotte's were common in Bloem, a university administrator named Kate Marais told me; it would be better to stay and understand it than to run away. Despite the fact that nearly everyone in town would have a copy of Mandela's *Long Road to Freedom* next to their Bible at home, these older homeowners would have been indoctrinated in the National Party schools, watching the state-sponsored news that depicted *swart gevaar,* or "black danger." While there was a period, during the dawning of democracy, when everyone came forward just a little bit, Marais said, in places like Bloem, the average white folks are "retreating. They're going back into their homes with their electric fences and their TVs."

It's the children of the older generation, both black and white, that are still an open question. Those born after 1994 call themselves "born frees," and they're just hitting college, where they unshackle themselves from the ideas of their parents and bloom into thinking of their own. They're the first generation to grow up without knowing apartheid firsthand, and yet the stain of their parents' knowing seeps through, as does the desire to do better. All three of these qualities braided together in the UFS racist incident and its aftermath.

At UFS, about 20 percent of all students live in residences — like dormitories — for their entire academic career. Each "res" is segregated by gender and, until 2007, by race. Segregation wasn't the plan, though: it just worked out that way at UFS and on many other campuses throughout the fledgling democracy.

"After the democratic election in 1994, the university started with the desegregation of the residences, but that triggered a huge upheaval in the student community with riots and everything. Students had firearms and were dropping bricks on cars," said W. P. Wahl, assistant director of UFS in charge of residence life. To keep the peace, the university allowed students to choose where newly admitted students were placed—and they chose to house along strict racial lines. But in 2007, when the born frees were thirteen and the current college students barely remembered apartheid, a new student council decided to try desegregation again. They called it the "transformation project."

Students at one residence rebelled. They lived at Reitz House, a Dutch-colonial-style male res with an inner courtyard and exposed dark wooden rafters. The transformation project brought 8 black students to live among the 128 white men, with the promise of more integration to come. Four white men rose up in protest with a video.

"Once upon a time, the Boers had fun living on Reitz Island," a student says in Afrikaans as the camera pans the Reitz bungalows and yellowing lawn. "Up until the day when the previously disadvantaged found the word 'integration' in the dictionary." The four white students, dressed in shorts and T-shirts, bring out five black cleaning staff, dressed in uniforms, to participate in a kind of "fear factor" game show, with a bottle of whiskey as the prize. The workers race down a track (which is later set to slow motion with "Chariots of Fire" playing in the background), dance to music in a hall, and awkwardly toss a football back and forth. At one point, unbeknownst to the workers, a student prepares a bowl of stew, and urinates into the bowl. He then serves it to the workers, who eat it off the dirt ground on their hands and knees. A final frame reads, "At the end of the day this is what we think of integration!"

The video was posted to Facebook and then to YouTube, and then went viral internationally. The four boys were put under criminal investigation, and the campus erupted in riots; students demanded the Reitz res be shut down for good. National papers as well as the *New York Times, Guardian,* and CNN all reported the debacle, all wanting to know: what was happening to Mandela's dream of a rainbow nation?

For me, watching the video from the States, it wasn't the racism that was surprising but the university's subsequent response, which was actually infused with a Mandela-like generosity, infused with ubuntu. I've taught at universities on both coasts over the past fifteen years, and I imagined that an incident like this would bring uproar and outrage against the students individually—they would be pilloried as bad apples in an academic barrel of good intentions.

"The biggest mistake made in the analysis of Reitz is to explain the incident in terms of individual pathology," said vice-chancellor and rector Jonathan Jansen in his inaugural address. Jansen was hired to run the university after the video, the first black rector in the university's history. "The question facing us, therefore, is a disturbing one and it is this: what was it within the institution that made it possible for such an atrocity to be committed in the first place?"

Claiming the Reitz Four were "children of this country, youth of this province, and they are students of the university," and that he could not deny them any more than he could deny his own children, Jansen withdrew all university charges—and in fact welcomed them back to complete their studies. It was a gesture, he said, of racial reconciliation and a need for healing. The five workers in the video were compensated.

This gesture, however symbolic (the students never returned and were charged in a criminal court), was a type of grand empathy I've never encountered in my years of teaching. Of course, the context in South Africa is entirely different; Mandela's spirit of reconciliation still serves as a guiding principle in both political moments and in smaller, everyday exchanges. It's hard to grasp the power of his hold on the nation—we don't have the same visionary figure here to bind us. More than once people asked me if I thought that if Martin Luther King hadn't been shot, American attitudes would be more united and generous today, but it was hard to imagine any figure occupying the American imagination the way Mandela does. There are statues and images of him in every city; nearly every home has a copy of his book; people reference him casually in conversation as a moral touchstone.

I also wondered about Jansen's insistence on collective action, another recurring South African theme, as a way to sidestep individual pain. Rather than closing the Reitz House down for good, he decided to turn it into an Institute for Studies in Race, Reconciliation, and Social Justice, as Jansen said, "a model for racial reconciliation for all students." Starting right then, all residences would be mandated to integrate with a 60/40 black/white ratio and, to help the first-year students expand their consciousness beyond the confines of race relations in South Africa, he instituted a freshman study abroad program.

I arrived on the campus six years after these promises — enough time to usher in an entirely new round of students who had no institutional memory of the video but were still fresh enough to feel its effects. I wanted to see if some mandated and difficult action — like integration — was possible if it was rooted, theoretically, in empathy. Jansen's idea wasn't to separate and punish students who had different, and even violent, ways of thinking. His idea was to welcome them in, understand them, and reconcile — and to spread this notion campus-wide. The question was, six years later, had it worked?

UFS IS A BEAUTIFUL CAMPUS. Creamy white Dutch-style buildings with pitched tile roofs appear along curved pathways beside blocky, 1970s architecture. Groundspeople tool around in golf carts tending to the many gardens, and students carry bright umbrellas to block the sun. You hear different languages everywhere — the soft clicks of Xhosa, the lulls and trills of Sesotho, the harder sounds of Afrikaans. While the government pays for all fees and books, it doesn't cover living expenses, so there are visible class differences. White students, generally, are behind the wheels of cars, parking at the lower lots. All students dress more modestly than in the United States, with longer skirts and more button-down oxfords. Everyone wears brighter colors. I did notice, as I got to know them, a few African students rotating the same two outfits day in and day out—a consequence of working long afterschool hours to pay for rent and food, with little left to spare.

Residences, generally speaking, don't cost more than off-campus housing, so rich are housed with poor, black with white, in the twenty-seven residences scattered about among the academic buildings and farther out near the athletic fields or main roads.

Each res has its own unique identity—they're more like our Greek system, with symbols and songs and, up until Jansen arrived and abolished them, initiation hazing rituals, than they are like dorms. Since UFS was an Afrikaans university, all of these old residence traditions were Afrikaner ones—and they had to be abolished if everyone was to feel welcome. But residence life, with its deep pride and cultural history, was integral to UFS; wiping out traditions was no easy task. The director of residences, W. P. Wahl, had to come up with something to replace them.

"We initiated what we call a cultural renewal process," Wahl told me. He is white and studious-looking, with thinning hair and rectangular wire-rimmed glasses. He comes from a ministry background, and his contemplative nature is clear. In every residence, Wahl said, they initiated a series of conversations about shared values—and from that developed new symbols and behavior patterns. "Your identity does not reside within your traditions. Your identity resides within your shared values, so if you make that switch, you're able to change the traditions."

"We're known as the res for pretty ladies," said Amukelani Khumalo, when I asked her about her residence, Welwitschia, whose symbol is a Namibian desert plant. But what about all the shared values Wahl had talked about? "Well, we have responsibility, respect, integrity," Amu ticked off. "And like, we use them to identify ourselves."

But did these terms work toward the desegregation Wahl and Jansen wanted so badly to achieve? Amu sighed and looked to her friend, another Welwitschia girl in a tracksuit and diamond stud earrings who was fiddling with her cellphone. They brought me into the residence lobby, a large, tiled room painted peach with a piano in the corner and metal armchairs clustered in groups of three and four.

"We have a culture day where we discuss all those diversity things and they [the administration] really do try and bring us together, but see it's not that easy because you're brought up to be white and we're grown up to be black," Amu said. Aside from its reputation as "pretty," Welwitschia is known as a white res; Amu told me that of the incoming seventy-five freshmen, fourteen were black and one was Indian. I came to learn that this was true of almost all the residences; despite the fact that the current ones are mandated to admit newcomers in roughly equal ratios, these newcomers know the reputations and accept at those that match their race. Thus segregation continues.

I did, however, find one res that just achieved racial parity with its incoming class. It's called Kestell, and I met with a girl on its residence committee named Erin Buys, proudly wearing her royal purple Kestell polo. Erin is coloured, a term used in South Africa to signify people of mixed-race, Malaysian, and Khoisan ancestry. Her mother, she says, has a hard time making friends outside of her coloured community. She worked in a bank under apartheid, as a teller, where strict race regulations kept her from moving up to management with the whites, and also from the back of the bank, where the blacks worked. Erin was born one year shy of being a born free and has had to struggle against her mother's belief that she's "belittled by white people and a little bit superior to black people."

This is an obvious shorthand for one experience in South Africa's long, embittered, and very complicated racial history, and I sensed Erin's resistance to oversimplifying. Still, any conversation about race can easily devolve into platitudes or broad statements in an effort to sweep people into neat camps for reconciliation. Erin's dividing lines cut along age.

"Really, you shouldn't focus on the seniors, don't waste your energy on that," Erin said, waving her hand in the air. Erin was a sophomore, and the seniors, she thought, were beyond saving. Kids just a few years younger, however, they had hope.

"I was born in '93, though I went to school with people who were born in '94. I've been able to witness the people who were born before the time, and obviously their parents had a much stronger influence. For myself and people younger than us, we also came from interracial schools already. We're used to it," she said.

Amu and her friend in the athletic gear, Reneilwe, came from integrated schools and are the same age as Erin—they'd been at UFS for a year. They both tried, they said, to make friends with the white kids when they first arrived but were rebuffed too many times. This gets exhausting, and the experience gets ingrained, and pretty soon, you just stick to your own.

"Why should I keep trying when you don't reply to my hellos? I'd rather just pass," Reneilwe said. "Just meeting someone and getting a hello back is not going to cure the world."

Erin understands this attitude and experience; it's the reason that, despite the mandate for racial parity, students choose residences associated with one racial bloc or another. "In my first year, we were called a black residence, just to be honest," Erin said, explaining that of her incoming class of forty-five girls, only five were white. But now that these younger girls have taken the reins of the residence committee, they've changed things. She noted the acceptance ratio the subsequent year was precisely half black and half white. The key to this change, Erin said, was language, and one-to-one connections.

"We worked very hard in getting the new first years to come, calling them, making them feel welcome. I'd speak to them in Afrikaans, for instance, I wouldn't speak to them in English, just to make them feel comfortable. We spoke to them in English, Afrikaans, Sesotho, and even IsiZulu," Erin explained. In the dorms themselves, they'd make sure to mix black and white; at dances, they'd play Sokkie music and R and B together; on specific cultural days, the girls could present songs or food from their backgrounds.

But then—and this is key—the girls would sort of forget about it. Individual cultural pride had its place, Erin said, but shared living conditions had to remain somewhat neutral territory. "We're not going to put up a Zulu sign, an Afrikaans sign. We're not going to erase [your heritage]. We're going to remember it in our heads and at the same time not even going to know it," she explained. "We'll do these little functions now and then where we celebrate it and embrace it but we're not going to advertise it to such an extent that it's almost like activism."

This idea of eliminating symbolism as a platform for beginning connections was interesting to me. (In the United States, where notions of individual rights and pride trump concepts of dignity and communality, I find we are saturated with symbols.) It's an idea that was echoed on the university's larger stage at the annual Reconciliation Lecture—held (symbolically) in the old Reitz Hall.

The hall was packed the year I visited, in 2015. Vice-Chancellor Jansen and Professor Gobodo-Madikizela were dressed in full robes to give introductions, and students from the music school sang opera. The guest lecturer was a man named Colm McGivern, a former student activist in Belfast, Ireland, at the height of the "troubles." McGivern wouldn't try to teach a South African audience anything about "the pain of liberation," he said—they knew that all too well —but he did say that the key to the Good Friday Agreement, which brought peace to Northern Ireland in 1997, "was to keep people apart, keep them away from each other."

In Northern Ireland today, McGivern said, "it's entirely possible for a young person to pass through their school days and not meet another person from another religion. Their first encounter is at university." As in South Africa, this puts a tremendous pressure on the institutions to "engage with that, deal with that phenomenon, or suffer the consequences."

The way McGivern's public school, Queen's University, engaged was to develop a slogan. Everyone, McGivern said, was to gear themselves toward "a neutral working environment." "It's an awful phrase, isn't it? Neutral working environment. But very powerful in its realization," he continued. "It was about creating a place of study . . . that was neutral in relation to its symbols and traditions."

Looking around the room, I wondered if UFS, a traditionally Afrikaner school in an Afrikaner state, could ever neutralize its territory. They had already changed a res name from Verwoerd (a South African prime minister when apartheid was entrenched) to Armentum, which is Latin for a herd of animals. But statues of apartheid-era heroes still remained dotted about. The audience that night was predominantly black — the effort toward, and interest in, reconciliation was one sided. This was a complaint I heard again and again.

"You can just look in terms of the students attending our events, and by far the black students are more interested," said J. C. van der Merwe, the deputy director of the institute — which had recently dropped "race" from its title and become, simply, the Institute for Reconciliation and Social Justice. Van der Merwe said that in South Africa, race is implied in any social justice act or gesture. "We really have to put in an effort to get white students interested."

When I met with van der Merwe at the institute, he was deep in a "Say No to Racism" campaign that was launching the next morning. Signs and posters emblazoned with the slogan were scattered all over his office, to be posted early before the school day, and he kept hopping up to answer the phone. The plan was to get students to pledge their adherence to the campaign online, stamp their thumb-prints on a giant banner, and wear wristbands in solidarity—and most important, attend antiracism discussions. Small-group conversations are a cornerstone of the institute, and they're backed by deep theoretical grounding.

The institute was launched by Bishop Desmond Tutu in 2011, and that same year, the organization published a forty-page research framework to shape the work of the institute going forward. It's called "Shared Complicities; Collective Futures," and it's a rich and complex document, referencing dozens upon dozens of philosophers —from Martin Heidegger to Gilles Deleuze, and a lot of Theodor Adorno, Judith Butler, and Slavoj Žižek.

The framework is too dense to summarize, but there are several points relating to empathy in a high-conflict zone that I find useful in many contexts. One is this notion of "mutual recognition": we tend to think of this as a common-sense goal in interactions, especially empathic ones; we believe we want to be mutually recognized when encountering the other. But André Keet, the primary author of the framework, takes the idea apart. Keet cites G. W. F. Hegel and his contention that mutual recognition is a source for a just society (a basic concept that we see adapted in the United States in everything from courtrooms to classrooms), and says instead that mutual recognition is a politics of the ego, an idea from Claudia Leeb. In other words, the desire to "mutually" recognize is really a desire to *be* recognized, "which violently suppresses difference." Keet says this urge toward mutuality actually leads to injustice, "since it rejects that which does not fit into the wholeness it defends." He leans toward something much less certain, citing Jacques Lacan, and says that we should look toward a kind of "subject-in-outline" rather than a subject in full knowability.

Like democracy, mutual empathy or understanding is always in the *becoming* and never in any kind of actualization. This idea, to me, is a relief—it moves us out of the static and into ongoing change, which is always where we are anyway. And this idea connects to another highly flexible conceptualization of reconciliation — that which Keet calls spectrality or hauntology.

Keet evokes the story of Louis Althusser, the French Marxist philosopher who strangled his wife to death in 1980. After he was arrested, Althusser was denied the right to stand trial by reason of insanity — in other words, he was denied the right to be guilty. This right, Keet asserts, is constitutive of being human. He was doomed to a kind of *spectral* existence, or as Althusser said, "neither dead nor alive, still unburied."

By extension, Keet says, those who were complicit under apartheid as perpetrators, but particularly as bystanders or beneficiaries, are also doomed to this spectral existence because they too are not allowed to be guilty. This gets back to the notion of the "little perpetrator" inside all of us and, Keet says, to Hannah Arendt's notion of banality: we are all, to varying degrees, guilty of perpetuating, or benefiting from, large systemic injustice — but to the extent that we're not called out on our own evils and held accountable (and who can be accountable to it all?), we are spectral, not fully alive or real.

Spectrality allows us to think about what is literally haunting the space when we try to reconcile — or even empathize — with anyone. Meaning: there's always more in the room, and, perhaps, something wanting to escape. Spectrality allows us to imagine what's disowned, unintegrated, not yet fully humanized — the guilt and culpability in ourselves and in the other.

These ideas of the other as spectral or in outline, to me, mean that any effort to empathize should, ideally, be undertaken with a light touch. If, as Keet says, "there are no neat boundaries between victims, perpetrators, beneficiaries, and bystanders" (and I would argue this is true in any communicative exchange), then any productive interaction wouldn't seek the fixed lines of rational, mutual understanding but rather a blurrier, shiftable goal. Perhaps empathy is merely mutual vulnerability.

. . .

FOR THE INSTITUTE, this exhaustive thinking and reasoning are the source of social action, lining up with Rector Jansen's mandate to the university to assign more meaningful cause to racist acts and response. But how does such theory resonate with the students themselves, who are living in a tense daily environment?

"Students don't want to intellectualize," said Nandi Bester, an honors student in international relations who did research with the institute. I met with six institute students one afternoon in the small, sunny scholars' room, with desks and a few computers against all the walls and backpacks littered about. In one of the institute's series of dialogues about the languages in which classes are taught, Bester said, students lost patience. "Students found they couldn't stand listening to theory when all they want to do is be able to apply the law to their own lives, their own personal lives."

The South African Constitution designates eleven national languages; the university utilizes three, though classes are held only in Afrikaans and English. A line in the national Bill of Rights reads, "Everyone has the right to receive education in the language or languages of their choice in public educational institutions where that education is reasonably practicable ... taking into account (a) equity; (b) practicability; and (c) the need to redress the results of past racially discriminatory laws and practices." Many African students claim the Afrikaans classes constitute discrimination because they cater to a smaller population and offer more individualized attention: the English classes are overcrowded, and students are forced to sit on the floor. They want the university to switch to English only; after all, they too must master a second language, as they're not offered classes in isiXhosa or Sesotho, for instance.

In other parts of the country, though, education for blacks and whites is even less equal, especially at the primary and secondary school levels. In poorer areas, books and supplies are not being delivered, and long-promised new schools stall in various stages of partial construction. People told me stories of meeting for classes under trees, and there are many news reports of people burning down existing schools in frustration.

"If you take the context nationally of what South Africans turn to to resolve our issues, you see underlying violence," Bester said. She thinks the institute is more than just a place to talk about specific problems at UFS. "The institute is a model to use to resolve conflicts, a platform for constructive dialogue."

But getting people to understand the importance of dialogue, the students told me, is an enormous undertaking, even just within the context and problems of the university. "We can't say we want to reunify the campus because that's assuming we were unified at one point. We're actually trying to build unity and conciliation, not reconciliation," said Phiwe Mathe, who the year before had been president of the student representative council. "That places a great expectation on the institute, that's what makes it such a slow process."

Mathe said that when a violent or racist incident occurs on campus, people want to talk about the precipitating events rather than the deeper causes. This makes sense to me: I think about how in the United States we can focus on tangible and concrete racist police violence more easily than the structural and historic racism that bred it.

The students at the institute that day were feeling somewhat discouraged. Even on the eve of their "Say No to Racism" campaign, violence from the previous year was overshadowing it, and, as Bester said, "the negative effects always seem to last longer than the positive highs."

The year before, two white students tried to hit a black student with their car and then beat him up while shouting racist slurs. The students were expelled. They faced attempted murder charges but were later found not guilty. While I was visiting the campus, these two students sent a letter claiming the university had harmed their reputations and demanding 1 million rand in damages.

"The institute is always in line with the vision of Professor Jansen to try and look at the deeper causes," Mathe said. But with such a volatile story, students weren't interested. "They don't want to look at what led to it all becoming so combustible in the first place."

Also, as everywhere, it's the daily micro-aggressions that wear people down and flatten their hope for participating in something like the institute. At first, Mathe said, most black students want to assimilate "because they think that assimilating will restore the peace, the harmony, and they don't want to disrupt anything. But then more and more incidents happen when it actually hits them that you're not actually being accepted here."

Even though they're in the minority percentage-wise, it's the Afrikaner students who assume the position of being able to accept or reject: because they have the historical precedence, they assume the position of power. "It's a culture of entitlement," Mathe said, and all of the conciliation efforts "make them feel as though they're being targeted, like something's being taken away." This can make some white students hold on tighter, or go on the attack, and black students "just disconnect from the space."

So how can you really hope for empathic dialogue from such disparate groups if you can't even get them to the table? I talked with Nyakallo Scheepers and Dintwa Serumula, the former and current presidents of the university's Golden Key, the Honour Society that recognizes the top academic achievers internationally. They were ostensibly two of the smartest students in the school. They both wore button-down oxfords and dark jeans, and spoke softly and swiftly. In terms of building empathy, they said, it wasn't just about bringing students to the table but changing the room the table was in.

Like so many other students I spoke with, Serumula lamented the classroom splits into Afrikaans and English—but not only because the Afrikaans classes provided better opportunities. He said the division meant black and white students could run their entire academic careers without really encountering the other.

"You need to create an environment where it will be easy for us to interact," Serumula said, which would happen if all courses were held in English. "You don't need to facilitate the process of reconciliation. Just increase the odds of us having a conversation."

The second part of building an empathic environment for reconciliatory dialogue is to recognize why certain parties disengage. At UFS, friction doesn't occur just along racial lines but socioeconomic ones. Something like 65 percent of the student body is food insecure. While the university is trying to soften this somewhat with food programs, this situation "places us in totally different worlds" from students who drive cars and have time for intramural sports, Scheepers said. It also leads to discouragement with the reconciliation process as a whole.

"It's been twenty-plus years since democracy; why do we still talk about reconciliation?" Scheepers asked, voicing the frustration students feel with the national promise that reconciliation would lead to equality. Serumula put it plainly: "We're walking every day and the majority of white students have cars. They managed to accumulate all this wealth, and we barely have enough money to last the whole month. We're at a disadvantage."

Scheepers nodded. "The socioeconomic barrier impedes reconciliation."

I told them that from my perspective coming from the United States, where we've had democracy for much longer and haven't achieved anything close to economic parity on any campus, twenty years seemed like a blip. Scheepers and Serumula agreed, but they had recently done an exchange program with the William Winter Institute for Racial Reconciliation at the University of Mississippi and pointed out a key difference.

"Here in South Africa I think we have a less volatile situation than there [in the U.S. South], where the heritage is too strong. With the younger generation, the attitudes they're inheriting — that process isn't interrupted, whereas here, it's always interrupted,"

Serumula said. He meant that in South Africa, blacks were continually gaining power because numbers were on their side. On a Mississippi campus, he saw "it was easier for whites to oppress the other people because they have nothing to lose."

So while both Serumula and Scheepers believed there was more impetus for change on a South African campus than an American one, they were surprised to see Confederate flags and memorial statues on a campus that housed a place like the Winter Institute. The physical environment, after all, sets a kind of stage for potential connections.

"They said there was a law that you couldn't change the monuments in Mississippi," Scheepers said, shaking his head. I pointed out that, walking around UFS, I stumbled upon a statue of C. R. Swart, the first president of South Africa, who served from 1961 to 1967, replacing the British monarch and governor-general as head of state. Swart was a fascist and a Nationalist (the party that launched apartheid). The university paid so much careful attention to the symbolic names of buildings, I wondered why they didn't erect more visually unifying imagery. Well, Scheepers conceded, even if UFS were to erect a statue of Mandela, for instance, "it could look like someone just placed it there to say, 'Okay, now, we're fine.' Which we're not."

ONE AFTERNOON, I met with Pumla Gobodo-Madikizela in a large public park filled with fifty or so bronze statues, all human-size, all marching in the same direction. I had flown across the globe to glean her insights on empathy, and she had chosen to meet me here: the symbolism wasn't lost on me. The monument is slated to be filled with four hundred heroes from the struggle for South African liberation and will, when it moves to its final home in Johannesburg, be the largest parade of statues in the world; at the back of the march are kings from the 1600s; at the front, leading everyone, will ultimately be Mandela.

Gobodo-Madikizela is petite, with quick, intelligent eyes and strong cheekbones. She favors bold necklaces and kitten heels; she carefully maneuvered her way on the grass around the statues, recognizing most of them by face. She stopped at Shaka Zulu, with his classic enormous shield and javelin. A mother was explaining to her daughter that this was a great Zulu king; the five-year-old touched the spear shyly.

"Remember that show?" the woman asked Gobodo-Madikizela. She was referring to the Shaka Zulu TV series that aired in the 1980s based on the historical novel by Joshua Sinclair.

Gobodo-Madikizela smiled and said of course; everybody watched it. Then she amended: "Well, all black families did."

In the 1980s, of course, white kids in school were being indoctrinated with Afrikaner history and politics. I asked Gobodo-Madikizela how the standard schoolbooks were being rewritten to reflect the garden where we were standing. The rewriting wasn't the trouble, she said. "The problem is, at the white schools, the white students aren't interested in this. They're only interested in their history."

Gobodo-Madikizela's solution was to write two history books, one Afrikaner and one African, that were stitched together and met in the middle. She said they do this in Israel and Yugoslavia. The book, I thought, would be a concrete symbol of what Nyakallo Scheepers suggested—rather than forcing reconciliation, it just would increase the odds of having a conversation.

But Gobodo-Madikizela thinks people need to be pushed a bit to empathize with the other—otherwise they don't leave the comfort zone of the familiar. "People are very much about being self-protective, about guarding their own interests," she said. She claimed she feels empathy for the white people she's encountered—on campus, in her prior work with the TRC, and simply in everyday interactions—who don't want to stretch into a fuller understanding of South African history.

"It doesn't mean I condone that thinking, but I have empathy because they have not transcended that place where they feel the deepest sense of loss," she said. "When you're faced with not only your actions but the losses of another, you have a perspective on history that says my gain was that person's loss."

And why would we, would anyone, *want* to feel another's loss? "Because that's what allows you to be self-reflective," she continued. "And reflection is necessary because that's the best way we can connect to others."

In the year after I left UFS, the institute continued its slow and important dialogue work, but another kind of conversation started happening too. Maybe students didn't think change was happening fast enough. Students, alongside workers who went on strike against jobs getting outsourced, began protesting a range of issues: the language policy, ongoing racism, and fee hikes. Property was damaged; some students were arrested. The school suspended classes for a week. In February 2016, demonstrators marched onto a rugby field during a game, and white spectators attacked the black protesters in a terrible show of brutality. By May, Rector Jansen had stepped down. But the university had announced an English-only policy for 2017.

As I followed the news from afar, I kept thinking of what Nyakallo Scheepers said to me about empathy being a way to interrupt power. Of course, I thought, but so was violence. That statue I had seen on the campus of the apartheid president C. R. Swart ended up hacked from its pedestal and ditched in a pond by the law school.

11

Empathy for the Enemy

When I went to South Africa, the face of apartheid — the man the press called "Prime Evil" — had just been granted parole, and the country was ablaze with the news. Eugene de Kock was originally condemned to two life sentences plus 212 years for crimes against humanity. De Kock was in charge of apartheid's notorious "C10" death squad, which captured, tortured, and murdered suspected anti-apartheid activists. All told, de Kock had eighty-nine counts against him — including six counts of murder, alongside attempt to murder, kidnapping, assault, illegal possession of firearms, and fraud. Beyond his personal murder count, he oversaw countless more, and he was vicious in his own attacks. When he found, for instance, an African National Congress activist gasping for life after an ambush he had ordered, he shot her twice in the head and pushed her car down a hill.

Pumla Gobodo-Madikizela's most famous book was about the time she spent with de Kock; she wanted to understand how a previously moral person could be brought to do such heinous acts, and she wanted to see if she herself could come to forgiveness. Gobodo-Madikizela had advocated for de Kock's parole; in the wake of the event, she too was all over the news.

"I found a man who was unmistakably tortured by his past, and by that I mean a man who was . . . confronting his deeds not as a cog in a machine but as a person who had done the deeds himself and was feeling very much remorse," Gobodo-Madikizela said on a South African radio program after the parole was announced. Remorse, for Gobodo-Madikizela, is a key part of forgiveness — which can only come on the heels of empathy. First, she argues, there's a component of "caring for" that goes beyond simple mirroring or feeling the other's pain in traditional definitions of empathy. In victim-perpetrator encounters, if the perpetrator feels remorse, this caring-for attitude can begin to kick in inside the victim, which in turn opens her to forgiveness.

But forgiveness may sound limiting, when in fact it is a kind of opening up. "People think when you forgive it means forgive and forget; in that case forgiving is the wrong word," Gobodo-Madikizela said on the radio program, adding that in South Africa, the word has come to represent a range of responses and meanings. "When we use the word 'forgiveness' we use it to say 'I no longer see you as the monster or the evil person who did these evil things to me or my family. I can now engage with you as a fellow human being.' It opens the door for another relationship to the traumatic past."

I went to South Africa in part to see for myself if this was true — and how it worked in real life. Gobodo-Madikizela wasn't the only one to meet and forgive de Kock; several of his victims' family members had done the same. And while the talk radio stations paraded angry voices demanding de Kock serve his time, most everyone I talked with agreed he should be released.

I wanted to understand how this was possible, how a man who had come to symbolize *prime* evil in a country beset with it throughout apartheid's terrible years could also be a symbol for empathy and forgiveness. Was it all symbolic, gestural, and therefore flimsy or false? Gobodo-Madikizela talks about turning acts of private empathy into public empathy, and de Kock's parole may have been the grandest such transformation of them all: the justice minister said he released him to the larger world because he was satisfied the families had been consulted. (Another apartheid criminal, Clive Derby Lewis, was not granted parole, in part because he didn't show "remorse.") I wanted to understand how the private matter of personal accountability toward one's victims could become a public forgiveness of the monster in everyone's mind, perhaps a kind of collective relief. The TRCs, for example, were public affairs, and communities could watch as individuals exchanged stories in an effort to extend the healing from the one to the many. And de Kock's stories of repentance were widely reported and disseminated. Again, collective healing seemed to be based on one-to-one exchanges.

To begin, I thought, I'd have to meet victim and perpetrator directly. The victim side was easier; a daughter of one of the men de Kock had murdered was coming to give a talk at the university where I was stationed. De Kock himself was being kept hidden for his safety (even his release date was a secret), but I did meet with someone who worked right under him, at apartheid's death squad prison, known as Vlakplaas. I thought he could give me insight into both the person and the conditions that came together to create Prime Evil.

"We were all evil," John said to me simply, from behind the wheel of his van. He drove now, for a living, ferrying tourists along the four- or five-hour journey from Johannesburg to various safari spots inside the massive Kruger National Park. He was in the army for the requisite two years and in the police force for fourteen, working in C10 under Eugene de Kock, though now he just lists the army service on his resume. He asked that I change his name. John was never called in before the court or the Truth and Reconciliation Commission, and though he acknowledges that de Kock was evil, he also sees him as something of a hero, for taking the hit when others wouldn't. "He took his sentence and told people where the graves were, and made peace with them. Some people got called in and said, 'No, it wasn't me.' It takes a man to admit what you did."

This is another reason Gobodo-Madikizela and others have

advocated for de Kock's release: keeping him behind bars would encourage what she calls "the great Forgetting." He becomes the one bad apple that's been put away and done with. Releasing him, she's written, humanizes him, and the more he's humanized, "the more we are forced to conclude there were factors that led him to do what he did. One must then ask, what were those factors?"

John agrees. He believes de Kock was a scapegoat and says all the political heads, including then-president F. W. de Klerk, knew what was happening at C10. (In an interview with BBC Radio, de Kock also said de Klerk's hands were "soaked in blood" and that he could name specific killings that he ordered.) De Klerk himself claimed to have a clean conscience and never stood trial for gross human rights violations.

"They knew about it but there was no paperwork; they never sent a handwritten or a typewritten order telling you to take someone out and interrogate him and then blow him up," John said. "This way, nobody could question you in court."

In the TRC hearings and in private meetings with families, de Kock exposed what the absent documents never could: he told the families how their loved ones had died and where the remains were buried. In this way, ironically, a perpetrator, or enemy, can help a victim heal. "They [victims' families] carry a lot of guilt," Gobodo-Madikizela told me — for not being there when the victim died, for not being able to intercede, for not knowing what even happened. "This person is transforming them back to the moment when they could not be present and [allowing] them to be there. So the perpetrator is helping them to work through their guilt."

When I asked John if he had faced, or would ever face, any of the families of his victims, he stalled. He wouldn't talk about whether he had killed anyone, though he said he tortured people and also that he remembered everything. "Your memory is a recording, there is no erasing, and certain smells, like the smell of diesel, will bring it all back," he said.

We were driving through the Drakensberg Mountains, a shockingly beautiful range of flat-topped crags, skirted in emerald and jutting into the sky, the tourists happily snapping pictures at the back of the van. Women sold mangoes and homemade beer at the edge of the road, and John quietly told me stories of his time in C10, a vein pulsing tensely at the side of his neck. It was clear the stories were painful. "You interrogate a guy, you give him an electrical shock or tie a jupe over the face so he can't breathe; the next time you take it a bit further," he said. As an example of something else, he described the way they used to train dogs to attack by setting them loose on the inmates, trapped in the yard. "You joke about it with your mates, and you're drinking so much, you just keep going."

This was enough evil for me. This was the closest I'd probably ever get to a paid state torturer, and I asked John how he could sleep at night. It was war, he said, and you had a war mentality. Which was a group mentality. You believed the propaganda that said the other side was a communist menace out to sell drugs to your kids. But really, the group-think started earlier than this.

"It was the way we grew up—you don't ask questions in church or in school," John continued. He was a bulky man, with a blocky head and soft, doughy features. He wore new black Converse high-tops and grey jeans. His smile, when it appeared, was shy and sweet, but his eyes were sad. John was raised to be a cop, like his father; education, he said, was for rich people. In high school, he learned first about the red menace, which transformed into the black menace—students were told the anti-apartheid activists were a communist underground threatening the very fiber of their country.

In the early 1990s, John said, this facade began to crack: "You can be macho and not feel, but when you lie on your own in bed, you start questioning things." For the most part, you didn't talk about what you did during the workday; John couldn't even tell his wife. So you drink more, and spend more time with your coworkers, who understand. "You get so used to seeing blood and dead bodies, you think it doesn't bother you, but it does. It's not normal."

Now, John says, many of his former colleagues are still drinking too much brandy, still living out the war in their heads, hanging out with one another and in chat rooms. He wishes that the state, after serving up so much propaganda, had also come up with some way to deprogram their former fighters in the years after democracy. John himself was deeply depressed and suicidal as he faced the lies that he'd been told and the truth of what he'd done.

John went to a private doctor to manage the depression, and stopped drinking, but he couldn't talk to his old comrades who couldn't admit their crimes. One on one and in small groups, he's talked with others about the torture he inflicted and says he feels "quite lucky to be strong enough to make peace with it."

But John didn't seem like a man at peace. He said he had no friends, save for his wife. He lived his life simply and carefully, driving the van most days, deep into the countryside where he could clear his head, and attending a black church on Sundays. He said he no longer trusted white people.

What gives John the slim measure of equilibrium in his life, unlike others he knows, is that he blames the government for some part of his past behavior, but not for everything. This is similar to de Kock, who has said repeatedly that he himself pulled the trigger. Like de Kock, John feels remorse.

"It's not that the government made us do it; you can't think that way," John said. "They made us not ask questions, they told us what to think, but also, we did it."

I WONDER IF John would feel more peace if he had made a public declaration of responsibility to the TRC or found his victims' families and talked to them directly. Then again, maybe peace isn't the point. Anyone who's met de Kock has said that he seems tormented, and perhaps that's an accurate leveling for what he's done. And even if John doesn't find or face accusers directly, when he talks with others who have been harmed by apartheid, it can have a vicarious effect, Gobodo-Madikizela says.

Gobodo-Madikizela writes about a useful "empathic unsettlement" that happens with secondary witnesses. She says that trauma testimonies can help people like John's old comrades, who are still longing for the war in their minds, and, to a different degree, the majority of white South Africans who benefited from apartheid but won't acknowledge their own accountability in the system. Essentially, she says, such people are yearning for "refuge in a simplified and stable version of the past." But since such a past never existed, they're forced to split, denying the reality of what was for this fantasy of what they wish had been.

This kind of splitting, of course, is something we're all capable of, and do, whenever we're nostalgic. Essentially, we block out our shameful, guilt-ridden memories—or externalize them by blaming others—like our parents, or the state, or systems of racism. Gobodo-Madikizela comes from a staunchly psychoanalytic stance, and she says the problem with nostalgia is that it short-circuits mourning—for what you did, for how others suffered—and if you cannot mourn, you cannot feel the edges of things, cannot hope for any meaningful, empathic reconciliation dialogue.

So, she says, secondary trauma statements can help shake loose, and reintegrate, those split-off parts. The other's testimony begins to butt up against our own stories from the past—the times we did or didn't take action for or against a victim—and our own guilt and shame are suddenly in an internal dialogue with the other. This itself is a kind of internal reconciling, and it's another reason de Kock, in the new South Africa, is better outside prison than in. When the minister of justice released de Kock, he said it was "in the interests of nation building." Behind bars, he's a criminal. Outside, he's one of us.

. . .

When Eugene de Kock killed Candice Mama's father, she was just eight months old. She grew up never knowing the details of her father's death — sometimes resentful of her father's absence, sometimes beyond furious at her father's killer. When Mama was twenty-three, de Kock reached out to her family; he wanted to say he was sorry. While Mama was nervous about the encounter, prison authorities tried to impress upon her what news outlets would later claim when he sought parole: de Kock was actually just a "normal man."

Mama's mother, grandfather, and two brothers all made the trip to the Pretoria prison, where they were first counseled by a chaplain and a therapist who served them tea and scones, alongside the prison director and a few guards. Mama told this story to a room full of students and faculty at the University of the Free State a few months after her visit. She's a poised college student who sat at the front of the room, graceful in her yellow blazer, flared dress, and ballet flats. "There's something about being told he's a normal man that kind of freaks you out because if he was so normal, why would you have to tell me?"

When de Kock finally came in, Mama said, she was surprised that trumpets didn't blare, she'd been waiting so long to confront him. But he just shuffled up to each person and shook hands, turning his good ear to hear them say hello.

More than anything, Mama said, de Kock wanted to provide her family with the opportunity to ask questions. He had been through these interviews before, and he knew people wanted to know details about their loved ones' last moments. Mama's father, Glenack, was a twenty-five-year-old activist who was murdered alongside four others in their car under a bridge in Nelspruit, a town in the northeast. Glenack was the driver. De Kock described emptying forty-seven bullets into Glenack's body and then planting arms and weapons and bombs into the car to make it look like an ambush. They then blew the car up, with all the dead passengers inside.

"He went into such elaborate detail of the encounter, at some point I was like, okay, that's enough," Mama said. Her mother wanted to know why de Kock targeted her husband, to which he said he had no valid answer. This, for Mama, was a kind of humility, and a key to her forgiveness. "He showed, 'It's not the system that made me do it; I did it. I'm the one that pulled the trigger,'" she said. Mama's question was whether he felt betrayed by the regime. "He said, 'Look, yes, I was working under this government but at the end of the day I'm the one who could have backed out at any moment and I continued to do what I knew was wrong.'"

Mama said she felt a lot of pressure to hate de Kock; the media depicted him as Prime Evil, and her own internal meter had told her for many years that a specific man had stolen her father from her. But the man she met, she said, was very broken. He had been under orders to murder and yet he felt a deep need to wrest that responsibility onto his own back. There's a certain way, when someone takes accountability for something they themselves can't even explain, that "they're not being condescending, but they're also not expecting you to understand. That's when you can cross over that boundary and say, 'I'm sitting across from another human being,'" she said, adding that she could feel his authenticity in his gestures, the look in his eyes. "It's just a natural thing. You rise up and understand him as a human being, rather than from a place of what society says you should do."

Gobodo-Madikizela says that we have multiple internal selves churning and chatting beneath one singular exchange with another. So when Mama the twenty-three-year-old heard de Kock take responsibility for his crimes, for instance, the thirteen-year-old inside her heard it too. "There is a dialogue not only on the outside with him in terms of words, but there is a dialogue with internal others," Gobodo-Madikizela said. "We're not encountering a person only in the external aspect of what we are; we carry things from the past. Our history, our memory of what happened. What your people did to me, what my people have suffered."

It's when these "internal others" get activated and start to reformulate their own histories based on the exchange with the other that transformation is possible. "Empathy is not something that happens just like that; there are so many small steps," Gobodo-Madikizela said, explaining that "the way you look at me, the way I see you, your vulnerability" are all "subtle" forms of communication beneath the words that also speak to the internal selves and help them shift. She told me, by way of example, the story of a white man she knew whose car had broken down in the karoo, a great swath of largely uninhabited desert. While he waited for help, a van full of black people pulled over. The man was scared they would rob him or hurt him, so he waved them on. Many hours later, it was night, and not another car had passed. The van came rumbling past again, this time from the opposite direction. The man grabbed his tire iron for protection as the van slowed; he hid it behind his back. But the people in the van had brought him soup and bread and water; they worried that he'd still be out there, and that he'd be hungry. Suddenly all the stories the man carried inside about robbery and danger, the younger selves that told him to be careful and wary, softened. Now, Gobodo-Madikizela says, the man works to create dialogue between people who formerly mistrusted one another.

It's a simple story but instructive for the process that happened with Mama. Once she met de Kock, the multidimensional man, he could no longer be the singular force of evil who had existed only to kill her father. In response, her frozen or fixed internal selves became more flexible too. "Usually trauma holds a person in a particular way — in a place of sadness, or a place of anger and hatred and resentment of others," Gobodo-Madikizela said. "What emerges in these encounters is they remember their pasts differently. Not to say they've jettisoned the memory but now there are different kinds of associations with the memory."

The prison allowed Mama's family about an hour with de Kock, and at one point, Mama said, she even cried for him, which confused her. It wasn't when he told her about losing his wife and sons, who left him when they found out what he'd done and who he'd been, though he told this story simply enough and without self-pity. It was when she asked him her second question and de Kock himself cried that Mama couldn't help herself.

"He's a very stoic man, very structured—he doesn't move, doesn't show emotion," Mama told the audience who had come to hear her speak. Everyone there knew what de Kock looked like from his endless pictures in the media: a tall, white man with a barrel chest and large, egg-shaped head. Thick, square glasses dominate his face, and he wears his straight brown hair brushed forward; his mouth is a thin, grim line. "He wiped the side of his eye, a tear was running down, and he said, 'You know, every time a family comes to see me the one thing I pray they never ask me is that question.'"

Mama had asked de Kock if he could forgive himself. He said he couldn't. "When you've done the things I've done," he said to Mama, "how do you forgive yourself?"

It is often easier for us to forgive another person than it is for us to forgive ourselves, and as Mama witnessed this universal experience playing out individually through de Kock, he joined the human race. "It's a strange thing, because this person becomes a human," she said. This echoes one of Gobodo-Madikizela's core beliefs, which is that to empathize is simply to humanize. "They feel what you feel, they go through what you go through, they're not this thing."

THE QUESTION, THOUGH, is why? Why would you *want* to empathize with someone who had killed your father? Why would you hope to humanize the enemy? I don't use the term "enemy" lightly here; I mean to signify the person or people who have committed such gross acts of violence or sadism they test the very limits of human compassion. There are whole bodies of literature, primarily Holocaust scholarship, that claim even trying to understand perpetrators of evil is an obscenity because evil acts cannot or should not be understood, and also because understanding can lead to forgiveness, and mass atrocity should never be forgiven.

Part of the answer, for Gobodo-Madikizela, Mama, and many others, is that the evil was not just rooted in one man. He lived and operated within a system of repression and atrocity, and as long as people continued to isolate and demonize him, they wouldn't look to the many others who were also accountable. Humanizing de Kock, in other words, widens the lens for other "evil" human beings to step into view. The other part of the answer is that if you don't reconcile the trauma through some form of transformation, Gobodo-Madikizela says, the trauma is bound to repeat itself. Her institute is currently studying second-generation trauma—the proliferation of rapes, a reinstitution of public murders in the townships, and, more broadly, xenophobia and deep economic injustice, which she describes as "at the bowels of the problem in our country."

Gobodo-Madikizela worries that a second violent uprising could occur—this time not between races directly, but between the rich and the poor, as the division becomes more stark and intolerable. She says that second- and third-generation post-apartheid South Africans expected their parents and grandparents' lives to be bleak but can feel increasingly betrayed that they're not currently reaping more benefit from the new, democratic system. Conversely, white families can feel that opportunities that used to be secure for their children are no longer givens. Lots of people believe that their options and promise are diminished in some way—a reason for the uptick in both crime and xenophobia. Gobodo-Madikizela believes that, rather than avoid conversations with the enemy or relegate them to the work of the past TRC, these discussions need to be fostered. She writes, "Listening to one another and acknowledging the experience of loss on both sides would be a start."

The final reason to engage with the enemy is one of real moral compunction. Since the enemy is not one but many, the question becomes how to live together and move forward. "When they acknowledge wrongdoing and show remorse, what should our response be? Should we reject their apology and continue to punish them with our hatred?" Gobodo-Madikizela asks. "Or should we extend our compassion and invite them to journey with us on the road of moral humanity?"

Compassion and care are important elements of Gobodo-Madikizela's definition of empathy. Sometimes, when meeting with an enemy—say, someone who killed a family member—you end up *wanting* your enemy to reclaim his humanity, because then your loved one didn't die in vain. "It's that caring dimension of empathy that's very important and often missed," she said. "It goes beyond stepping into the other person's pain; it's also caring for them."

Mama called her time with de Kock one of the most authentic exchanges she'd ever had, and I wonder if it was because of this: she entered the meeting expecting to get answers, perhaps an apology, but she didn't expect to leave feeling care and responsibility toward him too. It's the caring aspect of empathy that Gobodo-Madikizela says leads to social justice: Mama ultimately advocated for de Kock's parole.

As for forgiveness, for Mama, that really had very little to do with de Kock personally: she had forgiven him long before she even met him. As a young teenager, she said, she was angry—at Eugene de Kock and also at the world in general for depriving her of a father. She told herself that all the daily teenage frustrations in life wouldn't be happening if only she had a dad to talk to. She became, in her words, "an awful person to be around." But then, slowly, she realized her anger wasn't going to dissipate on its own. In order to become closer to her dad, she had to educate herself about the circumstances of his death.

So Mama read—about apartheid, about de Kock, about anything she could find about the day her father was murdered. At first, she considered de Kock a crazy man, and she resented him. But she found the resentment and continued anger were blocking her from having a happy life, from being, as she said, "a source of light." So in her mid-teens, and with de Kock nowhere in sight, Mama forgave him.

"Forgiveness was really a selfish thing," Mama explained. She felt she had to do it for her own health: she was sixteen and had ulcers; she went to bed angry, she woke up angry; she was miserable all the time. She thought a lot about what her father would have wanted her to do. "If my dad had been alive, would he have wanted me to be angry? Would he want me to sit here thinking, 'Oh God! If I find that man who did this I will kill them!'?"

Gobodo-Madikizela conceptualizes forgiveness as mourning the loss of revenge, and in a way, this is what Mama had to do. "You have to do the inner work to decrease that pain," Mama said, noting that even when justice is served, or revenge is meted, the anger doesn't go away. After all, de Kock was serving multiple life sentences, and Mama was still furious. "You must remember that letting go of your anger doesn't mean that you love your loved one any less."

Mama said that understanding that de Kock wasn't a lone operator helped her on her path: she knew he was under orders to kill. She said she also turned to God and trusted in a kind of benevolence greater than herself. The relief that came from forgiveness was worth it; Mama spent the latter part of her teenage years much freer and happier inside. The ulcers went away.

Forgiving de Kock a second time, in person, was easier. She simply said, "I forgave you then and I forgive you now." But this time, her forgiveness was laced with a real empathy for the man himself. Whereas her act of forgiveness was "selfish," she felt de Kock's urge to help families put their stories together was altruistic: nothing he did moved him closer to forgiving himself. "You can see where the person is broken, and yet they put aside their brokenness to assist you," she said. "This was a human being whose whole world was crushed. Imagine at thirty, forty, fifty, doing your work because someone says it's right. And then all of a sudden you just wake up one day and you don't have the foundation to justify everything you've done. You've just done bad."

RUMOR NOW HAS IT that Eugene de Kock will be relocated to Namibia; even though many South Africans feel as Mama and Gobodo-Madikizela do, he still likely wouldn't be safe living openly in his country. Like John the van driver, he'll live far away from his old haunts at Vlakplaas, but deep within his memories of everything he did there.

John says his own memories are like a tape that can't be erased, but also that he's processed them enough, and felt enough contrition, that he's confident he could never commit crimes again. He told me this as we drove through a small village in the foothills of the Drakensberg Mountains. Children kicked up dust at the side of the road; houses made of tin glinted in the sun behind them. Ahead of us, the asphalt was scorched with the telltale signs of burned tires, and I thought immediately of Gobodo-Madikizela's investigation into the ways trauma repeats itself when it hasn't been properly transformed. In apartheid days, people in the townships would "necklace" supposed apartheid sympathizers by throwing a burning tire around them. People were now burning ghosts—empty tires to protest the government's failed promise to build them a school.

Afterword

LOVE, A FUTURE

As I write this, back home in the States, it's hard to believe anybody's claim that empathy is gaining ground in our collective conscience or behavior. The number of hate groups and crimes have increased since Donald Trump's election: white nationalists mobilize violently in the streets, mosques receive letters advocating genocide, spray-painted swastikas appear on playgrounds, and teenagers shout "Build the wall!" at volleyball games. The war in Syria grinds on as our fear of migrants, terrorism, and the "other" rises to a furious pitch. England has left the European Union, we're threatening mass deportations, and, more locally, cops externalize this fomenting racism as they continue to shoot unarmed black men on the streets. It's hard to believe that empathy is winning.

And still, very recently, Hillary Clinton appeared on CNN imploring white people to "put themselves in the shoes" of black families. The chief of the Los Angeles Police Department called for recent police academy graduates to conjure more empathy. And a team of developers at the University of Southern California just built a virtual-reality video game for people to experience life at war in Aleppo, replete with bombs and refugee centers, precisely to generate more empathy for the Syrians surviving it. Empathy is certainly in the room, but is it, as some claim, the house we now live in? Have we entered, despite all the violence, the empathic era?

Jeremy Rifkin, in his book *The Empathic Civilization,* says that we have. Rifkin is an economic and social theorist from the Wharton School of Business, so he hails from the corporate universe invested in promoting empathy as the model for promoting sales. He draws on the Parma discovery of mirror neurons as proof that we are "soft wired not for aggression, self-interest, and utilitarianism," but rather for "sociability, attachment, affection, and companionship." He says our first drive is "to belong, and it's an empathic drive."

Upon this biological essentialism, Rifkin builds a narrative of four civilizations. Rifkin says that in hunter-forager societies, communication only went as far as a person could shout, so empathic ties extended along blood lines. Script came along with the second civilization, the hydraulic agricultural civilization, and people began to forge their ties along religious lines rather than the smaller tribal ones. Their sense of affiliation was growing. The third civilization was the Industrial Revolution, which collected human beings into nation-states, and suddenly people could extend their sense of belonging even further. Now, with the advent of the internet, Rifkin claims, we've entered an empathic civilization, where we can sense our membership in, and allegiance to, an entire planet. He cites things like the mass international response to the earthquake in Haiti as evidence of this newly expanded identity. His book is part history, part manifesto, as Rifkin contends that if we *don't* follow our natural, inborn imperative to be empathic toward an ever-developing family of humans, our planet is doomed.

I can easily, of course, counter Rifkin's utopic vision with myriad evidence of rising nationalism and religious fundamentalism. I can look abroad to Syria, where weaponized hate has triggered xenophobia in multiple countries, cast a glance toward Brexit, and then land back home, where a galvanized political movement is based on building a wall to keep others out.

I could argue that we're a planet steeping in bigotry, increasingly stalwart in its political nihilism, but I'm not a historian and it's so difficult to get the long view and predict a future when trauma-tized by current events. One philosopher who does is Luc Ferry, and he comes to an almost opposite conclusion to Rifkin's. Ferry argues that, in the West, we've gone through five major eras (he's quite Eurocentric in his scope), each defined by a different "principle," or framework, for the meaning of life. Ferry says we're becoming ever more interior, rather than expansive, in our outlook. It's not the era of empathy we've just entered, Ferry argues, but the Era of Love.

The first principle Westerners followed, in the era of the early Greeks, was what Ferry calls the Cosmological Principle, where the aim was to move from the initial chaos of life to the harmony of the cosmos. In the Greek conception, we lived in a hierarchal world where everyone had his assigned place, and our salvation was a kind of anonymous return to the natural order. In the next era, from the end of the fourth century through the seventeenth, religion domi-nated Western thought and salvation became personal; one attained it through God and faith. The next principle was humanist, and it extended through the Enlightenment. In this period, Westerners bet their salvation more on human accomplishments—like building and science—and people themselves were the new heroes. Time speeds up for Ferry as the next principle, the Deconstruction Prin-ciple, came in with Arthur Schopenhauer and bloomed with Fried-rich Nietzsche, who proclaimed that God was dead. In this era, we began to think that we could no longer judge life from the outside because we were living inside it, that there was no longer anything to aspire to but life itself. Salvation, Ferry says, wasn't to be found in transcendence but in immanence.

The final principle, where we've landed currently, is the Prin-ciple of Love, which is what now gives meaning to our existence. It's a kind of second humanism, but one born from changes in family structures. It was only after the Second World War that marrying for love became universal, first in Europe and then to a greater or lesser extent in the rest of the world, Ferry argues—and it's this radical shift in our personal lives that has radically shifted our public lives too. In the Middle Ages, marriage was based on biology, lineage, and economics. With the Industrial Revolution, people moved to towns and sought accommodations there, and young women especially had newfound freedoms. Marrying for love caught on with the working class first, and as these arrangements ceased to be purely economic, the notion of loving one's offspring blossomed as well. In the Middle Ages, for example, the death of a child was viewed often as less serious than the death of a pig or a horse. At the dawn of the nineteenth century, some 30 percent of children were abandoned. But now, we've entered an era where we expect all of our primary relationships to be rooted in love.

The risks of this change, Ferry says, are that we love our children so much that we don't prepare them for the wider world (he doesn't go so far as to say we spoil them, but that's the implication), and we build a culture where youth is lionized. Philosopher Alain Badiou writes that partnerships of choice are, with the internet, morphing into hyper-curated "safety-first" relationships, losing all the risk and adventure of real love. So this new era is not without its drawbacks.

But what are the broader, positive effects of this increasingly inward-gazing shift? In a way, they're the same as Rifkin's predictions, even as he claims we've become more global in our orientation. Because our primary drive is to create a life of love with spouses and children, Ferry suggests, our actions, politics, and art are geared toward future generations in a way they haven't been before. We're more interested in preserving the earth and building social institutions that protect the communities our children will inherit. In this way, his era of love lines up with Rifkin's empathic era: we're beginning to care about the other as never before.

I draw from these two thinkers because they both look at historical sweeps, at eras, rather than the smaller units of decades or years. And when we soften our eyes to the larger picture rather than scrutinize the daily violence, maybe what they're saying is true. Again,

I'm not a historian, but I do know, from my research and experience with this book, that while humanity may be moving along an arc toward more empathic- or love-based societies, the practice of moving from the specific to the general is still just that: we don't love or empathize with whole communities because we want to; we don't forgive a genocidal state until we first have one-to-one interactions with the other. Only then can our imaginations expand.

I've thought a lot about the difference between love and empathy in the terrible months after I returned from South Africa and found my marriage wrenched apart, my capacity for imagining a future collapsed. The things Seth did were pedestrian, base, and very human, and so were my reactions. We were reduced to our limbic selves, rendered primal as he cheated and I raged, then he beat me and I ran, only to come back — desperate to cling onto the only life I knew. When I had some emotional distance from the pain, which was rare, I could feel empathy for Seth: he was subject to the storm toss of a new chemical, testosterone, that made him a stranger to himself. This empathy, I thought, was born of love. If he had been on chemo, which makes people foggy, or some other altering drug, I would already love him enough to empathize with his transgressions.

Some biological evolutionists make the opposite claim. Love, they say, was born of empathy, which is an older, more primitive instinct. Babies mirror this human evolution in their own development, as they can first empathize, imitating facial expressions or cries, and then move on to the more complex articulations of love. But this formulation accounts for only the simplest definition of empathy, that of mere mirroring, and not for the layered and nuanced empathic understandings I've come to adopt.

After all of this research, two of my favorite definitions are these: empathy is an interruption of power, and empathy is mutual vulnerability. Both definitions call upon an aspect of loving, and so I'm not sure which came first, the empathy or the love. I suspect they're braided together, are mutually reinforced.

I *am* sure, at the end of it all, that empathy's not a skill, like love is not a skill, though one can improve empathy's expression, the breadth of its reach. I've come to think of empathy as a moral art, which sounds like an oxymoron but is more of a paradox, if you hold it gently enough. Empathy, as art, can be genius and inborn, and as practice, be refined and improved. But it's also moral in that it's a way one chooses to angle herself rightly in the world, interrupting power, and remaining vulnerable, both. Just think of the empathy masters who deployed it in the hardest of circumstances, up against the wall of oppression—the Gandhis, the Kings, the Mandelas. They were practicing a moral art.

And this is how I got myself through. In the end, I found that being empathic to Seth's rage did interrupt the power it held over us both. Through empathy, I held the rage apart and found it toxic; whether it was endemic to Seth or to the substance he injected, it didn't matter anymore. Where once I had tipped the scales, in love, to empathize with Seth's plight over my own safety, mutual vulnerability called for a return to the self. I remember, for instance, seeing my face in the mirror after a bad fight. I had a black eye and a split lip; these things were non-negotiable evidence that he was powerless over his own fury, no matter what stories we told about it. And I had to see myself too; I had to tune in and take care.

At the beginning of this project, I thought self-empathy was self-indulgence, but I see now that it's the in breath that allows the out breath to occur. I thought, when I left Seth, that I'd be utterly alone, but what I found was that I returned to the world and that the world returned to me. Friends came forth, and I found a self that I had forgotten; I went inward and outward at once.

This mirrors, in the broadest sense, Ferry's forecast. When, as a people, we have moved more inward toward love, we also gaze outward toward a future for that love to take seed. And when we have empathy for the enemy outside, we can fold it back to the littlest tyrant within us all. This is, after all, my hope.

Acknowledgments

Primary thanks for this book go to the many, many sources who contributed their time and ideas, and whose stories are contained in these chapters.

I wrote *I Feel You* during a shocking and terrifying breakup, and many dear friends got me through and got me writing each day. I truly wouldn't be here if not for Teresa Dias, Dorla McIntosh, and Sam Feder—you are my family and my home. Deep thanks also to my sister-in-arms Sharon Krum and to Tracey Goodman, who loved me through. Carin Clevidence, thank you for your wisdom and your swimming skills, and Lisa Hanauer, I love you to the moon. Thank you to my dear friends Sara Ingram, Isabelle de Rezende, and Virginia Vitzhum, who kept me laughing, and to Carol Edelstein and Robin Barber, who kept the faith. Thanks to Emma Heaney for our long drives and deep talks. Thanks to Heart Montalbano, whose name says it all, and to Cindy Tolan, Jennie Yabroff, Kit Rachlin, and T Wilkins. Thank you also to M Burgess, who kept me open; Ilana Sharp from so very far away; and Lelena and Milo Azarmsa, who swept in and kept me sane. Thank you to Claire Hertz, for really everything. Finally, thank you to my brilliant and vibrant daughter, Christina, who teaches me about love and empathy every day.

Several dear friends read drafts of *I Feel You* or provided feedback on ideas as I went along. Alison Smith read early chapters and was an ongoing champion of the book. Meehan Crist and Ellis Avery spent long days writing with me and discussed many facets of the project. *I Feel You* is a better book for all of you, and I am deeply grateful. Thanks too to Atticus Zavaletta, who read a later draft and provided deep support and understanding, and to Gemma Baumer, who transcribed many of the interviews.

Andrea Schulz acquired this book and provided the initial framing ideas; I've never worked with a finer mind or a deeper spirit. I was beyond lucky to then land with Ben Hyman as my editor; Ben understood the essence of *I Feel You* in ways I didn't even see and pushed me to ask deeper, richer questions so the book became more dynamic and alive. Eamon Dolan then became the editor and championed this book up to the finish line; thanks also go to Margaret Hogan for her eagle-eyed copyediting. Amy Williams, my long-term agent and dear friend, has stood by me through all the hills and valleys. Thank you.

I Feel You would not have been possible without the incredible gift of time and space provided by several artist colonies and residencies. My deepest gratitude goes out to the MacDowell Colony, the Corporation of Yaddo, the Marble House Project, and the Virginia Center for the Creative Arts for providing me, and so many other artists, the place, and the faith, to do our work.

Notes

Introduction

page

xiv   *"I see your post"*: Josh Constine, "Facebook Is Building an Empathy Button, Not 'Dislike.' Here's How It Could Work," *Tech Crunch,* September 15, 2015, http://techcrunch.com/2015/09/15/the-sorry-button/.

     $5.84 billion a quarter: Everett Rosenfeld, "Facebook Smashes Street's Highest Estimates on Revs and EPS," *CNBC,* January 27, 2016, http://www.cnbc.com/2016/01/27/facebook-q4-earnings.html.

xv   *"Corporate Empathy Is Not":* Belinda Parmar, "Corporate Empathy Is Not an Oxymoron," *Harvard Business Review,* January 8, 2015, https://hbr.org/2015/01/corporate-empathy-is-not-an-oxymoron.

     in empathic design: Brianna Crowley and Barry Salde, "Building Empathy in Classrooms and Schools," *Education Week,* January 20, 2016, http://www.edweek.org/tm/articles/2016/01/20/building-empathy-in-classrooms-and-schools.html.

     "profit" of the classroom: Beth Holland, "Empathy, Strategy and Edupreneurship: Fostering a Culture of Innovation," *Education Week,* April 6, 2016, http://blogs.edweek.org/edweek/edtechresearcher/2016/04/empathy_strategy_and_edupreneurship_fostering_a_culture_of_innovation.html?_ga=1.227571609.503848817.1460055292.

1. The Sound of Science

3   *$800 million a year:* Acxiomcorp, http://www.marketwatch.com/investing/stock/acxm/financials.

4   *multiple fields:* Giacomo Rizzolatti et al., "Premotor Cortex and the

Recognition of Motor Actions," *Cognitive Brain Research* 3, no. 2 (March 1996): 131–141.

As Rizzolatti said: This was a taped interview. See Go Cognitive, interview with Giacomo Rizzolatti, http://www.gocognitive.net/interviews /initial-reaction.

"can explain many things": Ibid.

5 *precursors to such a process:* Vittorio Gallese and Alvin Goldman, "Mirror Neurons and the Simulation Theory of Mind Reading," *Trends in Cognitive Sciences* 2, no. 12 (December 1998): 495.

"expectations, and the like": Ibid.

start to lie: Chris D. Frith and Uta Frith, "Interacting Minds—A Biological Basis," *Science,* November 26, 1999: 1692–1695.

6 *another's emotion comes:* Amy Coplan and Peter Goldie, eds., "Introduction," in *Empathy: Philosophical and Psychological Perspectives* (Oxford: Oxford University Press, 2014), x–xi.

people like Thomas Hobbes: Jennifer A. Herdt, *Religion and Faction in Hume's Moral Philosophy* (Cambridge: Cambridge University Press, 1997), 24–29.

own self-interest: Internet Encyclopedia of Philosophy, s.v. "egoism," http://www.iep.utm.edu/egoism/.

entry for "somatic sympathy": Evelyn L. Forget, "Evocations of Sympathy: Sympathetic Imagery in Eighteenth Century Social Theory and Physiology," *History of Political Economy* 35 (2003): 292.

sympathies they evoked: A good book on this phenomenon and era is Ildiko Csengi, *Sympathy, Sensibility and the Literature of Feeling in the Eighteenth Century* (New York: Palgrave Macmillan, 2012).

7 *less occult-sounding terminology:* Forget, "Evocations of Sympathy," 295–303.

empathy again could bloom: Gustav Jahoda, "Theodor Lipps and the Shift from 'Sympathy' to 'Empathy,'" *Journal of the History of the Behavioral Sciences* 41, no. 2 (Spring 2005): 153.

into bodily ones: A good article on Lipps's theories of *Einfühlung* and its distinction from sympathy can be found in Jahoda, "Theodor Lipps and the Shift from 'Sympathy' to 'Empathy,'" 151–163.

experiencing a straightening: This notion of aesthetic empathy was furthered particularly by Vernon Lee in her famous book *Beauty and Ugliness,* originally published in 1912. Vernon Lee and Clementina Anstruther-Thomson, *Beauty and Ugliness and Other Studies in Psychological Aesthetics* (London: Andesite Press, 2015). A good article on this is Carolyn Burdett, "'The Subjective Inside Us Can Turn into the Objective Outside':

Vernon Lee's Psychological Aesthetics," *19: Interdisciplinary Studies in the Long Nineteenth Century* 12 (2011), https://www.19.bbk.ac.uk/articles /10.16995/ntn.610/.

8   *others understand us:* Coplan and Goldie, "Introduction," xii–xiv.

deeper feelings: Caitlin Dewey, "A Noted Philosopher's Argument for Signing Off Social Media . . . and Enjoying the 'Brief Time' You Have Left," *Washington Post,* June 4, 2014, https://www.washingtonpost.com /news/the-intersect/wp/2014/06/04/a-noted-philosophers-argument-for -signing-off-social-media-and-enjoying-the-brief-time-you-have-left/.

9   *mirror neurons "empathy neurons":* V. S. Ramachandran, "The Neurons That Shaped Civilization," TED India, November 2009, https:// www.ted.com/talks/vs_ramachandran_the_neurons_that_shaped _civilization?language=en.

only in the motor region: Christian Keysers, "Current Biology: Quick Guide: Mirror Neurons," *Cell* 19, no. 21 (November 17, 2009): R971– R973.

someone else being touched: Vilayanur (V. S.) Ramachandran, "Mirror Neurons and Imitation Learning as the Driving Force Behind 'the Great Leap Forward' in Human Evolution," *Edge,* May 31, 2000, https://www .edge.org/conversation/mirror-neurons-and-imitation-learning-as-the -driving-force-behind-the-great-leap-forward-in-human-evolution.

many of his claims: See links here for more scientific critiques: http:// www.wired.com/2013/12/a-calm-look-at-the-most-hyped-concept-in -neuroscience-mirror-neurons/.

10   *"rather dull and stupid.":* See Go Cognitive, interview with Giacomo Rizzolatti.

seen them in monkeys: In 2010, Roy Mukamel and colleagues at UCLA claimed to have found direct evidence of mirror neurons in humans with single-cell electrodes implanted in the brains of twenty-one patients with pharmacologically intractable epilepsy. Roy Mukamel et al., "Single-Neuron Responses in Humans During Execution and Observation of Actions," *Current Biology* 20, no. 8 (April 27, 2010): 750–756. Depth electrodes were implanted to monitor for seizures, and researchers asked these patients to do some experiments. The controversy here was that the researchers were constricted by clinical considerations (these were people, not monkeys), and electrodes were not implanted in the same regions as they were in the macaques. The implants included regions in the medial frontal cortex and the medial temporal lobe (the amygdala, the hippocampus, the parahippocampal gyrus, and the entorhinal cortex). If mirror neurons are everywhere, critics claimed, then they lose their explanatory power. In these experiments (which included grasping and facial recognition), neurons showed increased, decreased, and mismatched firing rates — a result that critics claimed discounted their status as potential mirror neurons.

anger in music: A great list of scientific articles linking mirror neurons to all kinds of human behavior can be found in Gregory Hickok, *The Myth of Mirror Neurons: The Real Neuroscience of Communication and Cognition* (New York: Norton, 2014), 24–25.

11 *insert their micro-electrodes:* Rizzolatti et al., "Premotor Cortex and the Recognition of Motor Actions," 132. The article refers to surgical procedures in a previously published paper: M. Gentilucci et al., "Functional Organization of Inferior Area 6 in the Macaque Monkey I. Somatotopy and the Control of Proximal Movements," *Experimental Brain Research* 71, no. 3 (1988): 476.

much smaller neocortex: Marco Iacoboni, *Mirroring People: The Science of Empathy and How We Connect with Others* (New York: Picador, 2009), 9.

12 *99 percent of our DNA:* Ann Gibbons, "Bonobos Join Chimps as Closest Human Relatives," *Science,* June 13, 2012, http://news.sciencemag.org/plants-animals/2012/06/bonobos-join-chimps-closest-human-relatives.

granted legal personhood: Thomas Rose, "Going Ape over Human Rights," CBC News, August 2, 2007, http://web.archive.org/web/20100203225450/http://www.cbc.ca/news/viewpoint/vp_rose/20070802.html.

thinkers in multiple fields: H. F. Harlow, R. O. Dodsworth, and M. K. Harlow, "Total Social Isolation in Monkeys," *Proceedings of the National Academy of Sciences of the United States of America* 54, no. 1 (July 1965): 90–97.

13 *psychologists like John Bowlby:* Harry Harlow and John Bowlby were in close personal communication from the mid-1950s through the mid-1970s and relied on one another's work. For an interesting discussion of their exchanges, see Frank C. P. van der Horst, Helen A. LeRoy, and René van der Veer, "'When Strangers Meet': John Bowlby and Harry Harlow on Attachment Behavior," *Integrative Psychological and Behavioral Science* 42 (2008): 370–388.

fraternities and social offices: Fred Rosenbaum, *A Social and Cultural History of the Jews of the San Francisco Bay Area* (Berkeley: University of California Press, 2009), 255.

poor breeding: Harlow studied under Lewis Terman. See Wikipedia, s.v. "Lewis Terman."

14 *"grossest profanity":* John M. Harlow, "Recovery from the Passage of an Iron Bar Through the Head," *Bulletin of the Massachusetts Medical Society* (1868), reprinted in *History of Psychiatry* 4, no. 14 (1993): 274–281.
    "you like monkeys?": Interview with *Pittsburgh Press-Roto,* 1974, quoted in Deborah Blum, *The Monkey Wars* (Oxford: Oxford University Press, 1994), 92.

15 *"alternating gender incongruity":* L. K. Case and V. S. Ramachandran, "Alternating Gender Incongruity: A New Neuropsychiatric Syndrome Providing Insight into the Dynamic Plasticity of Brain-Sex," *Medical Hypotheses* 78, no. 5 (May 2012): 626–631.

16 *"do little harm":* The full quote reads, "False facts are highly injurious to the progress of science, for they often endure long; but false views, if supported by some evidence, do little harm, for everyone takes a salutary pleasure in proving their falseness; and when this is done, one path towards error is closed and the road to truth is often at the same time opened." Charles Darwin, *The Descent of Man and Selection in Relation to Sex,* 1st edition (1871), chap. 21, "General Summary and Conclusion," http://www.gutenberg.org/cache/epub/2300/pg2300.html.

18 *"neither male nor female":* Tom Gardner, "'Our Gender Shifts by the Hour': Incredible Claim of Group Who Suffer from 'Phantom Genitalia,'" *Daily Mail,* April 20, 2012, http://www.dailymail.co.uk/sciencetech /article-2132793/Our-gender-shifts-hour-claims-group-suffer-phantom -genitalia.html.

20 *non-motor regions:* Researchers recorded extracellular activity from 1,177 cells in medial frontal and temporal cortices while the patients executed or observed hand-grasping actions—just like the monkeys in Parma. Patients also observed facial emotional expressions. Roy Mukamel et al., "Single-Neuron Responses in Humans During Execution and Observation of Actions," *Current Biology* 20 (April 27, 2010): 750–756.

2. Teach Your Children Well

24 *students thirty years ago:* Jamil Zaki, "What, Me Care? Young Are Less Empathetic," *Scientific American,* January 1, 2011, https://www.scientific american.com/article/what-me-care/.

25 *caring about other people:* This comes from an unpublished Making Caring Common Executive Summary, 2014, provided by Rick Weissbourd.

26 *emotion recognition software:* Raffi Khatchadourian, "We Know How You Feel: Computers Are Learning to Read Emotion and the Busi-

ness World Can't Wait," *New Yorker,* January 19, 2015, http://www.new
yorker.com/magazine/2015/01/19/know-feel.

our private messages: A book that discusses this concept thoroughly is Jim
Dwyer, *More Awesome Than Money: Four Boys and Their Heroic Quest to
Save Your Privacy from Facebook* (New York: Viking, 2014), esp. 44.

27   *among other topics:* Fifth International Workshop on Empathic Computing, program guide, December 1–5, 2014, Gold Coast, Australia, http://
www.ai.sanken.osaka-u.ac.jp/IWEC2014/.

Department of Defense: T. J. McCue, "Google's Motorola May Give You
a Tattoo or Vitamin Password," *Forbes,* June 5, 2013, http://www.forbes
.com/sites/tjmccue/2013/06/05/googles-motorola-may-give-you-tattoo
-or-vitamin-password/.

29   *programs are running:* Suzanne Bouffard, "Teach the Teachers Well,"
The Opinionator, New York Times Blog, April 30, 2014, http://opinionator
.blogs.nytimes.com/2014/04/30/teach-the-teachers-well/?_r=0.

30   *better grades:* See the Collaborative for Academic, Social, and Emotional
Learning's fact page on outcomes, http://www.casel.org/social-and-emo
tional-learning/outcomes.

31   *"empathy teaching program":* Roman Kzarnac, "Six Habits of Highly
Empathic People," *Greater Good,* November 27, 2012, http://greatergood
.berkeley.edu/article/item/six_habits_of_highly_empathic_people1.

35   *stages of empathy development:* Martin Hoffman's four stages of development are concisely explained at https://www.msu.edu/~mandrews
/mary/empathy.htm, citing H. R. Schaffer, *Social Development* (Oxford:
Blackwell, 1996).

38   *homeless people or war veterans:* Martin Hoffman, "Empathy, Justice, and
the Law," in Coplan and Goldie, eds., *Empathy*, 235–236.

39   *not a feeling:* See Dominic McIver Lopes, "An Empathic Eye," in Coplan
and Goldie, eds., *Empathy*, 118–133.

defendant was sad: O. Tsoudis, "The Influence of Empathy in Mock Jury
Criminal Cases: Adding to the Affect Control Model," *Western Criminol-
ogy Review* 4, no. 1 (2002): 55–67.

response and viewing time: L. M. Brown, M. Bradley, and P. Lang, "Affective Reactions to Pictures of Ingroup and Outgroup Members," *Biological Psychology* 71 (2006): 303–311.

plastic dinosaurs too: Tanya Lewis, "Humans Show Empathy for Robots,"
Live Science, April 23, 2013, http://www.livescience.com/28947-humans
-show-empathy-for-robots.html.

40   *essays on empathy:* Coplan and Goldie, eds., *Empathy.*

41   *"rational, western, masculine":* Nel Noddings, *Caring: A Relational Ap-*

proach to Ethics and Moral Education (Berkeley and Los Angeles: University of California Press, 2013), 30.

42 *"self-reliance/self-confidence"*: In Japan, 31 percent chose "sympathy/empathy/concern for others" as their top answer to the question "What are the most important things for children to learn in preschool?" In the United States, 34 percent chose "self-reliance/self-confidence" as their top answer to the same question. In each instance, these answers garnered the highest percentages out of eleven possible answers. There were three hundred total respondents according to an email interview with Joseph Tobin. Percentages come from Joseph Tobin, Joseph Y. H. Wu, and Dana H. Davidson, *Preschool in Three Cultures: Japan, China and the United States* (New Haven, Conn.: Yale University Press, 1991), 190.

"satisfy their wishes": T. S. Lebra, *Japanese Patterns of Behavior* (Honolulu: University of Hawaii Press, 1976), 38, as cited in Kazuya Hara, "The Concept of *Omoiyari* (Altruistic Sensitivity) in Japanese Relational Communication," *Intercultural Communication Studies* 15, no. 1 (2006): 27.

43 *maintained for three years:* In 2001, the Healthy Child Committee of Cabinet in the province of Manitoba commissioned a randomized, controlled study and follow-up study of the program. Researchers found that the ROE group had reduced aggression and improved prosocial behavior immediately after completing the program, and those outcomes were maintained or further enhanced over the three years after the program ended. Quoted from the Roots of Empathy website, "Report on Research, 2009," http://www.rootsofempathy.org/documents/content/ROE_Report_Research_E_2009.pdf.

3. The Experimental Self

44 *Molly:* Not her real name.

46 *Seth:* Not his real name.

48 *Sierra Leone:* Marshall B. Rosenberg, *Nonviolent Communication: A Language of Life* (Encinitas, Calif.: Puddledancer Press, 2003), 11.

54 *studies might conjure:* Patricia S. Churchland, *Touching a Nerve: Our Brains, Our Selves* (New York: Norton, 2013), 20.

landscape of our selves: Patricia S. Churchland, "Feeling Reasons," in Paul Churchland and Patricia Churchland, *On the Contrary: Critical Essays, 1987–1997* (Cambridge, Mass.: MIT Press, 1998), 232–254.

electric shocks: See William Wan and Xu Yangjingjing, "Gay Activists in China Sue over Electric Shock Therapy Used to 'Cure' Homosexu-

ality," *Washington Post,* July 31, 2014, https://www.washingtonpost.com
/world/asia_pacific/gay-activists-in-china-sue-over-electric-shock
-therapy-used-to-cure-homosexuality/2014/07/31/cd155d5e-18a9-11e4
-9349-84d4a85be981_story.html?utm_term=.ea5c4c4dbb9b.

56 *20 percent of the prison population:* Kent Kiehl, *The Psychopath Whisperer:
The Science of Those Without Conscience* (New York: Crown, 2014), 177.
schizophrenia, autism, or ADHD: Andrea L. Glenn and Adrian Raine,
Psychopathy: An Introduction to Biological Findings and Their Implications
(New York: New York University Press, 2014), conclusion, Kindle version.
do so violently: Kiehl, *The Psychopath Whisperer*, 25.

57 *federal prison inmates:* Stav Ziv, "Report: America's Prison Population
Is Growing Again," *Newsweek,* December 22, 2014, http://www.news
week.com/americas-correctional-system-numbers-293583.
average male is four: Kent Kiehl and Julia Lushing, "Psychopathy,"
Scholarpedia 9, no. 5 (2014): 30835, http://www.scholarpedia.org/article
/Psychopathy.
pure psychopathy: Kiehl, *The Psychopath Whisperer*, 49.
employment history, and so on: Ibid., 45–46.

58 *correlated with psychopathy:* For more specific data on this particular
study, see Elsa Ermer et al., "Aberrant Paralimbic Gray Matter in Criminal Psychopathy," *Journal of Abnormal Psychology* 121, no. 3 (2012): 640–
658.

61 *saw fear:* See Mark R. Dadds et al., "Attention to the Eyes and Fear-Rec-
ognition Deficits in Child Psychopathy," *British Journal of Psychiatry* 189
(2006): 280–281.
"social functioning": Mark R. Dadds et al., "Impaired Attention to the
Eyes of Attachment Figures and the Developmental Origins of Psychopathy," *Journal of Child Psychology and Psychopathy* 52, no. 3 (2011): 239.
Also, for a good overview of Dadds's work, see Michelle Griffin, "Bad to
the Bone," *Sydney Morning Herald,* September 20, 2011, http://www.smh
.com.au/national/bad-to-the-bone-20110919-1khts.html.

62 *default position:* "Brain Research Shows Psychopathic Criminals Do Not
Lack Empathy, but Fail to Use It Automatically," *Eurekalert,* Oxford
University Press, July 24, 2013, http://www.eurckalert.org/pub_releases
/2013-07/oup-brs071913.php.
brains lit up: Harma Meffert et al., "Reduced Spontaneous but Relatively
Normal Deliberate Vicarious Representations in Psychopathy," *Brain*
136 (August 2013): 2550–2562.

4. Ars Empathia

64 *full faces:* Kelly Servick, "Want to Read Minds? Read Good Books," *Science,* October 3, 2013, http://www.sciencemag.org.ezproxy.cul.columbia.edu/news/2013/10/want-read-minds-read-good-books.

65 *one week later:* P. Matthijis Bal and Martijin Veltkamp, "How Does Fiction Reading Influence Empathy? An Experimental Investigation on the Role of Emotional Transportation," *PLoS One* 8, no. 1 (January 30, 2013): http://journals.plos.org/plosone/article?id=10.1371/journal.pone.0055341.

schools in forty-six states: David Comer Kidd and Emanuele Castano, "Reading Literary Fiction Improves Theory of Mind," *Science,* October 18, 2013: 380.

66 *immediate and instinctive:* Jahoda, "Theodor Lipps and the Shift from 'Sympathy' to 'Empathy.'"

67 *"subjective experiences":* Kidd and Castano, "Reading Literary Fiction Improves Theory of Mind," 380.

"idea reaching out": Sontag is describing Roland Barthes here; see "Writing Itself: On Roland Barthes," in *A Susan Sontag Reader* (New York: Farrar, Straus and Giroux, 1982), 445.

68 *"hatred and despair":* James Baldwin, "Notes of a Native Son," *Notes of a Native Son* (Boston: Beacon Press, 2012), 115.

"had been cut": Ibid., 97.

70 *human eyes:* Traci Pedersen, "Attending Live Theater Boosts Empathy, Tolerance in Students," *Psych Central,* October 19, 2014, http://psychcentral.com/news/2014/10/19/attending-live-theater-boosts-empathy-tolerance-in-students/76308.html.

movement in our bodies: See "Watching Dance: Kinesthetic Empathy," which uses audience research and neuroscience to explore how dance spectators respond to and identify with dance. It is a multidisciplinary project involving collaboration across four institutions (University of Manchester, University of Glasgow, York St. John University, and Imperial College London). See http://www.watchingdance.org.

bumps the empathic response: Stacey Kennelly, "Does Playing Music Boost Kids' Empathy?" *Greater Good,* June 8, 2012, http://greatergood.berkeley.edu/article/item/does_playing_music_boost_kids_empathy; Jill Suttie, "Sharing Music Builds Trust, Empathy and Cooperation—Here Are Four Ways Science Proves It," *Yes Magazine,* February 4, 2015,

http://www.yesmagazine.org/happiness/four-ways-music-strengthens
-social-bonds.

71 *mass atrocity:* For a good description of some of these studies, see Cynthia
Cryder, George Lowenstein, and Richard Scheines, "The Donor Is in
the Details," *Organizational Behavior and Human Decision Processes* 120
(2013): 15–23.

5. Courting Empathy

84 *lifelong recidivism:* See, for example, Barry Holman and Justin Zeiden-
berg, "The Dangers of Detention: The Impact of Incarcerating Youth in
Detention and Other Secure Facilities," Justice Policy Institute, Washington, D.C., 2006, http://www.justicepolicy.org/images/upload/06-11
_rep_dangersofdetention_jj.pdf.

85 *consolidated lands:* Henry's two older brothers were given Normandy and
England, but Henry tactfully witnessed the death of one brother and
captured the other in battle and popped him in prison for life.

86 *adult counterparts:* The most comprehensive survey of victim mediation
programs comes from the year 2000, where researchers found 289 victim-
offender mediation programs in the United States. Of the 94 programs
that responded to the researchers' questionnaire, 45 percent worked only
with juvenile offenders and their victims, 9 percent worked only with
adult offenders and their victims, and 47 percent worked with both.
Mark S. Umbreit and Jean Greenwood, "National Survey of Victim-Offender Mediation Programs in the United States," Center for Restorative
Justice and Peacemaking, University of Minnesota, St. Paul, U.S. Department of Justice, Office of Justice Programs, 2000: 5.

89 *main offense:* Howard Zehr, *Changing Lenses: A New Focus for Crime and
Justice* (Scottdale, Penn.: Herald Press, 2005), 163.

90 *actions for restitution:* Molly Rowan Leach, "From Punitive to Restorative
Justice: The Call and Response," *Kosmos,* Fall/Winter 2013, http://www
.kosmosjournal.org/article/from-punitive-to-restorative-justice/.

91 *Angela's:* Not her real name.

93 *"empathy to play":* Jess Bravin, "'Empathy' Takes a Knock in Confirmation Hearings," *Wall Street Journal,* July 20, 2009, http://www.wsj.com
/articles/SB124804842579363835.
"lived that life": Wilmer J. Leon III, "Empathy vs. Ideology on the
Court?" *truthout,* June 4, 2009, http://truth-out.org/archive/component
/k2/item/84428:empathy-vs-ideology-on-the-court.

94   *"Obama empathy test"*: Bravin, "'Empathy' Takes a Knock in Confirmation Hearings."

    court decisions: Carol Lloyd, "Empathy's Poster Child," *GreatSchools,* August 3, 2016, http://www.greatschools.org/gk/articles/a-little-girls -passion-turns-the-whole-family-upside-down/.

95   *express sadness:* Jesse Prinz, "Is Empathy Necessary for Morality?" in Coplan and Goldie, eds., *Empathy*, 226.

96   *"cuteness effects":* Ibid., 226.

    than if he is not: Lee cites Jill D. Weinberg and Laura Beth Nielsen, "Examining Empathy: Discrimination, Experience, and Judicial Decision-making," *Southern California Law Review* 85, no. 2 (2102): 338–339, reporting the results of an empirical study using data from a large random sample of federal district court filings of employment civil rights cases between 1988 and 2003 in seven cities: Atlanta, Chicago, Dallas, New Orleans, New York City, Philadelphia, and San Francisco. The report finds that white judges ruled for the defendant employer on a motion for summary judgment in 61 percent of cases while minority judges did the same in only 38 percent of cases, and that this difference is statistically significant.

    level playing field: Rebecca K. Lee, "Judging Judges: Empathy as the Litmus Test for Impartiality," *University of Cincinnati Law Review* 82 (2014), http://scholarship.law.uc.edu/uclr/vol82/iss1/4.

97   *implicated in a case:* From Martha C. Nussbaum, *Poetic Justice: The Literary Imagination and Public Life* (Boston: Beacon Press, 1996), contending that "though empathy with the actors will usually be one important part of the process of judicious spectatorship, through which the judge takes the measure of the suffering of the people . . . the judicious spectator must go beyond empathy, assessing from her own spectatorial viewpoint the meaning of those sufferings and their implications for the lives involved." Cited in Lee, "Judging Judges."

98   *stayed low:* C. G. Lee et al., *A Community Court Grows in Brooklyn: A Comprehensive Evaluation of the Red Hook Community Justice Center* (Williamsburg, Va.: National Center for State Courts, 2013), 174–177.

    thirty-three in other countries: Ibid., 10.

99   *within the community:* Ibid., 3–4.

    "narrow-minded, and innumerate": Paul Bloom, "The Baby in the Well: The Case Against Empathy," *New Yorker,* May 20, 2013, http://www .newyorker.com/magazine/2013/05/20/the-baby-in-the-well.

100   *in terms of entanglement:* Lori Gruen, *Entangled Empathy: An Alterna-*

tive Ethic for Our Relationships with Animals (Brooklyn: Lantern Books, 2014).

6. Empathy Traffic

102 *undercut the empathy:* C. Daniel Batson et al., "Empathy and Attitudes: Can Feeling for a Member of a Stigmatized Group Improve Feelings Toward the Group?" *Journal of Personality and Social Psychology* 72, no. 1 (1997): 105–118.

relief or objective: Jill Bennett and Suzanne Keen have written powerfully about these concepts; see the introduction to Tim Gauthier's *9/11 Fiction, Empathy and Otherness* (Lanham, Md.: Lexington Books, 2015), 30–31.

103 *nation on earth:* The United States has the highest prison population rate in the world, at 716 per 100,000, as of the latest available data, October 2013. Roy Walmsley, "World Prison Population List, Tenth Edition," International Centre for Prison Studies, London: University of Essex, http://www.prisonstudies.org/sites/default/files/resources/downloads /wppl_10.pdf.

3,400 nationwide: National Institute of Justice, Drug Courts Information Page, http://www.nij.gov/topics/courts/drug-courts/Pages/welcome .aspx.

clinically dependent: "Alcohol, Drugs and Crime," fact sheet, National Council on Alcoholism and Drug Dependence, Inc., https://ncadd.org /for-youth/drugs-and-crime/230-alcohol-drugs-and-crime.

104 *"out of the life":* Sarah Schweig, Danielle Malangone, and Miriam Goodman, "Prostitution Diversion Programs," Center for Court Innovation, 2102, 3, http://www.courtinnovation.org/sites/default/files/documents/ CI_Prostitution%207.5.12%20PDF.pdf.

children are trafficked: Eleanor Goldberg, "Sex Trafficking Isn't an 'Over There' Issue, 100,000 U.S. Kids Are Sold into It Every Year," *Huffington Post,* November 2, 2014, http://www.huffingtonpost.com/2014/11/02/sex -trafficking-kids-us_n_6083890.html.

looking for them: See Carol Smolenski, executive director for ECPAT-USA, speaking in a public service announcement on trafficked kids in the United States, "It Happens Here," published October 29, 2014, https://www.youtube.com/watch?v=Xr0rv1zVZJ4.

105 *control of sex trafficking:* See Taryn Offenbacher, "Gang Sex Trafficking on the Rise," Shared Hope International, March 28, 2014, http:// sharedhope.org/2014/03/28/gang-sex-trafficking-rise/; "Street Gangs and Modern Slavery," *Global Centurion,* http://www.globalcenturion

.org/programs/researchanddevelopment/streetgangs/; and "Alleged Gang Members and Associates Indicted in Cross-Country Sex Trafficking Conspiracy," FBI press release, San Diego Division, December 11, 2014, https://www.fbi.gov/sandiego/press-releases/2014/alleged-gang-mem bers-and-associates-indicted-in-cross-country-sex-trafficking-conspir acy.

resources and help: "Changing Perceptions: A Conversation on Prostitution Diversion with Judge Fernando Camacho," research sheet, Center for Court Innovation, January 2012, http://www.courtinnovation.org /research/changing-perceptions-conversation-prostitution-diversion -judge-fernando-camacho-0.

106   *"18 years of age":* Office to Monitor and Combat Trafficking in Persons, U.S. Department of State, "Trafficking in Persons Report 2015," https:// www.state.gov/j/tip/rls/tiprpt/2015/243359.htm.

110   *discrimination on the job:* Brad Sears and Lee Badgett, "Beyond Stereotypes: Poverty in the LGBT Community," *TIDES/Momentum,* June 2012, http://williamsinstitute.law.ucla.edu/headlines/beyond-stereotypes -poverty-in-the-lgbt-community/.

111   *one's own benefit:* C. Daniel Batson, "The Empathy-Altruism Hypothesis," in *Altruism in Humans,* Oxford Scholarship Online, May 2011, http:// www.oxfordscholarship.com/view/10.1093/acprof:oso/9780195341065. 001.0001/acprof-9780195341065-chapter-2.

    expectation of reward: C. Daniel Batson, "Addressing the Altruism Question Experimentally," in *Altruism and Altruistic Love: Science, Philosophy and Religion in Dialogue,* eds. Stephen G. Post et al. (Oxford: Oxford University Press, 2002), 89–105.

112   *helping largely stopped:* Participants rated the extent of oneness they felt with the evicted person by responding to two items that were combined in all analyses to form a oneness index. The first item incorporated the Inclusion of Other in the Self (IOS) Scale used by Aron et al. to measure perceived self-other boundary overlap. A. Aron et al., "Inclusion of the Other in the Self Scale and the Structure of Interpersonal Closeness," *Journal of Personality and Social Psychology* 63 (1992): 596–612. It consisted of a set of seven pairs of increasingly overlapping circles. Participants selected the pair of circles that they believed best characterized their relationship with the evicted person. The second item asked participants to indicate on a seven-point scale the extent to which they would use the term "we" to describe their relationship with the evicted person. For purposes of counterbalancing, the oneness index items appeared either immediately after participants engaged in their description of the target

person or after all other measures were taken. From Robert B. Cialdini et al., "Reinterpreting the Empathy-Altruism Relationship: When One into One Equals Oneness," *Journal of Personality and Social Psychology* 73, no. 3 (1997): 484.

street-based prostitutes: Juhu Thukral and Melissa Ditmore, "Revolving Door: An Analysis of Street Based Prostitution in New York City," Sex Workers Outreach Project, Urban Justice Center, New York, 2003: 6, 10.

sexual labor: "New Study Shows 25 Percent of Homeless Youth Victims of Trafficking or Sexual Labor Before Finding Shelter at Covenant House," press release, Covenant House, March 9, 2015, https://www .covenanthouse.org/homeless-youth-news/new-study-shows-25-percent -homeless-youth-victims-trafficking-or-sexual-labor.

provide emergency housing: Molly Crabapple, "Special Prostitution Courts and the Myth of 'Rescuing' Sex Workers," *Vice,* January 5, 2015, https:// www.vice.com/en_us/article/sex-workers-and-the-city-0000550-v22n1.

overcrowded already: The number of homeless New Yorkers sleeping each night in municipal shelters was 78 percent higher in the fiscal year 2014 than it was ten years prior, according to "Basic Facts About Homelessness: New York City," Coalition for the Homeless, http://www .coalitionforthehomeless.org/basic-facts-about-homelessness-new-york -city/.

no cost to them: Steven L. Neuberg et al., "Does Empathy Lead to Anything More Than Superficial Helping? Comment on Batson et al. (1997)," *Journal of Personality and Social Psychology* 73, no. 3 (1997): 510–516.

113 *attorneys, and agencies:* Juhu Thukral, Melissa Ditmore, and Alexandra Murphy, "Behind Closed Doors: An Analysis of Indoor Sex Work in New York City," Sex Workers Outreach Project, Urban Justice Center, New York, 2003: 15.

114 *hands of the police:* See, for instance, "Policing Sex Work," Incite National, http://www.incite-national.org/sites/default/files/incite_files/resource _docs/4668_toolkitrev-sexwork.pdf, and Thukral and Ditmore, "Revolving Door."

been assaulted: Thukral and Ditmore, "Revolving Door," 7, 37–38.

16 percent of the population: See "Criminal, Victim or Worker? The Effects of New York's Human Trafficking Intervention Courts on Adults Charged with Prostitution-Related Offenses," Red Umbrella Project, October 2014, executive summary, http://redumbrellaproject.org /wp-content/uploads/2014/09/RedUP-NYHTIC-ExecutiveSummary Web.pdf, and Crabapple, "Special Prostitution Courts and the Myth of 'Rescuing' Sex Workers."

targeted people of color: In 2013, a federal judge ruled that the stop-and-frisk policies of the New York Police Department violated the constitutional rights of minorities in the city. About 83 percent of the stops between 2004 and 2012 involved blacks and Hispanics, even though they make up just over 50 percent of the city's population. Joseph Goldstein, "Judge Rejects New York's Stop-and-Frisk Policy," *New York Times,* August 12, 2013, http://www.nytimes.com/2013/08/13/nyregion/stop-and-frisk-practice-violated-rights-judge-rules.html?pagewanted=all&_r=1.

115 *"minutest incidents":* Adam Smith, *Theory of Moral Sentiments,* ed. K. Haakonssen (1759; Cambridge: Cambridge University Press, 2002), part 1, chap. 1, pp. 7, 35, as cited in Adam Morton, "Empathy for the Devil," in Coplan and Goldie, eds., *Empathy,* 323.

116 *other person's agency:* See Peter Goldie, "Anti-Empathy," in Coplan and Goldie, eds., *Empathy,* 302–317.

118 *empathy can increase:* Morton, "Empathy for the Devil," 318–330.
"rather than the immorality": Ibid., 327.

7. Performing Empathy

123 *made life bearable:* Eva Illouz, *Why Love Hurts: A Sociological Explanation* (Cambridge: Polity Press, 2012), 7–8.

127 *literature of testimony:* As cited in Shoshana Felman, "Education and Crisis; or, The Vicissitudes of Teaching," in Shoshana Felman and Dori Laub, *Testimony: Crises of Witnessing in Literature, Psychoanalysis and History* (New York: Routledge, 1992), 21.
"on all the testimony": Primo Levi, *The Drowned and the Saved,* transl. Raymond Rosenthal (New York: Simon and Schuster, 1986), 41.

128 *for the witness:* Paul Celan, "Ashglory," in *Breathturn into Timestead: The Collected Later Poetry, a Bilingual Edition,* transl. Pierre Joris (New York: Farrar, Straus and Giroux, 2014), 65.
way into understanding: Shoshana Felman writes about this idea of the fragmentary nature of testimony in Felman, "Education and Crisis," 20.

135 *spectrum of social stories:* Jo Salas, *Improvising Real Life: Personal Story in Playback Theatre* (Dubuque, Iowa: Kendall/Hunt, 1993), 5–15.

136 *transmuted into a story:* Ibid., 19.
mental health improved: Julie Beck, "Life's Stories," *Atlantic,* August 10, 2015, http://www.theatlantic.com/health/archive/2015/08/life-stories-narrative-psychology-redemption-mental-health/400796/.

8. Fall from the Tree

142 *more than thirty countries:* See Wikipedia, s.v. "Mindfulness-based stress reduction."

149 *mode of perceiving:* Gail S. Reed, "The Antithetical Meaning of the Term 'Empathy' in Psychoanalytic Discourse," in *Empathy I,* eds. Joseph Lichtenberg, Melvin Bornstein, and Donald Silver (Hillsdale, N.J.: The Analytic Press, 1984), 13.

put the emphasis there: Sullivan and Winnicott, for instance, both addressed empathy, but it was Kohut who really placed it front and center. See James S. Grotstein, "Some Perspectives on Empathy from Others and Toward Oneself," in Lichtenberg, Bornstein, and Silver, eds., *Empathy I,* 201.

152 *gratification and praise:* For more about the rise of this cultural creation of a narcissistic prototype, see Elizabeth Lunbeck, *The Americanization of Narcissism* (Cambridge, Mass.: Harvard University Press, 2014).

but too little: Ibid., 3, 59, 60.

157 *ingredient for empathy:* See Pumla Gobodo-Madikizela, "Psychological Repair: The Intersubjective Dialogue of Remorse and Forgiveness in the Aftermath of Gross Human Rights Violations," *Journal of the American Psychoanalytic Association* 63, no. 6 (December 2015): 1085–1123.

riddled with ambivalence: For more on this idea, see C. Fred Alford, "Forgiveness as Transitional Experience: A Winnicottian Approach," *International Journal of Applied Psychoanalytic Studies* 10, no. 4 (December 2013): 319–320.

158 *"gone missing as well":* Judith Butler, *Precarious Life: The Powers of Mourning and Violence* (Brooklyn: Verso, 2004), 22, as cited in ibid., 320.

9. State of Empathy

161 *placement in the country:* See "What Is the History," Maine-Wabanaki REACH, http://mainewabanakireach.org/what-is-the-history/.

in state custody: Ibid.

162 *REACH:* REACH stands for Reconciliation-Engagement-Advocacy-Change-Healing.

164 *"highnesses may command":* See Wikipedia, s.v. "Requerimiento."

non-Native kids to be removed: Lorie Graham and Kathryn E. Fort, "If Truth Be Told," *The Hill,* June 25, 2015, http://thehill.com/blogs/congress-blog/civil-rights/245996-if-truth-be-told.

166 *access to electricity:* Laurie Guevara-Stone, "Native Energy: Rural Electrification on Tribal Lands," *RMI Outlet,* June 24, 2014, http://blog.rmi

.org/blog_2014_06_24_native_energy_rural_electrification_on_tribal
_lands.

169 *"can strike its roots"*: Maria Popova, "Philosopher Martha Nussbaum on
Human Dignity and the Nuanced Relationship Between Agency and
Victimhood," *BrainPickings,* January 6, 2016, https://www.brainpick
ings.org/2016/01/06/martha-nussbaum-agency-victimhood-dignity/?mc
_cid=2985ffb498&mc_eid=8d6119c0ee.

177 *revoked their sovereignty:* Ramona du Houx, "Maine's Governor LePage
Rejects Tribal Sovereignty in Executive Order to Possibly Take Over
Fishing Grounds," *Maine Insights,* April 21, 2015, http://maineinsights.
com/currentmainenews/14139601/gov-lepage-rejects-tribal-sovereign
tyost.
legislature entirely: Colin Woodard, "Maine Tribes Will No Longer Recognize Authority of State Officials," *Portland Press Herald,* May 27, 2015,
http://www.centralmaine.com/2015/05/27/maine-tribes-will-no-longer
-recognizing-authority-of-state-officials/.

10. To Interrupt Power

179 *"who we all are":* This particular definition comes from Liberian peace
activist Leymah Gbowee.

180 *Charlotte:* Not her real name.
split 70/30: Jonathan Jansen, *Leading for Change: Race Intimacy and Leadership on Divided University Campuses* (New York: Routledge, 2015), 11.

183 *"the first place?":* From the Inaugural Lecture of the 13th Rector and
Vice-Chancellor of the University of the Free State, Professor Jonathan
D. Jansen, October 16, 2009, http://www.politicsweb.co.za/news-and
-analysis/why-were-withdrawing-charges-against-reitz-four--j.

190 *full knowability:* André Keet, "Social Justice, Reconciliation and Non-
Racialism, Shared Complicities; Collective Futures: The Research
Framework of the Institute (2012–2016)," University of the Free State,
Bloemfontein, South Africa: 10, http://www.ufs.ac.za/docs/librariespro
vider39/home-page-documents/executive-summary-of-the-research
-framework-1-eng.pdf?sfvrsn=0.

191 *"still unburied":* Ibid., 18, citing Louis Althusser, *The Future Lasts a Long
Time* (New York: New Press, 1992), 16.
fully alive or real: Ibid., 18.

192 *"laws and practices":* The Constitution of the Republic of South Africa, 1996,
issued December 2009, chap. 2, Bill of Rights, "Education."

193 *schools in frustration:* See, for instance, "South Africa Is Burning and

We Do Not See It," *My News 24*, May 5, 2016, http://www.news24.com /MyNews24/south-africa-is-burning-and-we-do-not-see-it-20160505.

1 million rand in damages: Sapa, "UFS Mullin R 1m Damages Claim," *IOL*, March 6, 2015, http://www.iol.co.za/news/crime-courts/ufs-mulling -r1m-damages-claim-1828110.

198 *classes for a week:* "Classes Set to Resume at UP, UFS After Protests," SABC News, February 29, 2016, http://www.sabc.co.za/news/a/e9495b 804bdb391697989796fb2bb898/Classes-set-to-resume-at-UP,-UFS-after -protests-20160229.

show of brutality: Alyssa Klein, "Black Student Protestors Beaten by White Students During University of Free State Rugby Match in South Africa," *Okay Africa*, February 23, 2016, http://www.okayafrica.com /news/university-of-free-state-south-africa-student-protestors-beaten -by-white-students-during-rugby-match/.

had stepped down: Mbali Sibanyoni, "Mixed Reactions to Prof Jansen Resignation," SABC News, May 16, 2016, http://www.sabc.co.za/news/a /b54532004cc905108540b7af52343cc3/Mixed-reactions-to-Prof-Jansen -resignation-20160516.

English-only policy for 2017: Shenaaz Jamal, "University of the Free State Dumps Afrikaans Lessons," *Rand Daily Mail*, March 15, 2016, http:// www.rdm.co.za/politics/2016/03/15/university-of-the-free-state-dumps -afrikaans-lessons.

11. Empathy for the Enemy

199 *down a hill:* Ali Mphaki, "Daughter of Victim Forgives de Kock," *IOL*, February 13, 2012, http://www.iol.co.za/news/crime-courts/daughter-of- victim-forgives-de-kock-1232693.

200 *parole was announced:* From an interview with Pippa Hudson on the radio program "Cape Talk," January 30, 2015. See "'Eugene de Kock: Tortured by His Past' — Former TRC Councillor," January 30, 2014, http:// www.capetalk.co.za/articles/1538/trc-councillor-on-eugene-de-kock -parole.

opens her to forgiveness: Gobodo-Madikizela, "Psychological Repair," 1110–1111.

201 *families had been consulted:* "Minister Michael Masutha: Parole Decision on Inmates Barnard, de Kock, and Lewis," media statement, South African Government, January 30, 2015, http://www.gov.za/minister -michael-masutha-parole-decision-inmates-ferdi-barnard-eugene -alexander-de-kock-and-clive.

202 *"were those factors?":* Pumla Gobodo-Madikizela, *Dare We Hope? Facing Our Past to Find a New Future* (Cape Town: Tafelberg, 2014), loc. 1211, Kindle edition.

killings that he ordered: Mohammed Allie, "Jailed Policeman Accuses de Klerk," BBC News, July 27, 2007, http://news.bbc.co.uk/2/hi/africa/6919569.stm.

205 *secondary witnesses:* Pumla Gobodo-Madikizela, "Remembering the Past: Nostalgia, Traumatic Memory, and the Legacy of Apartheid," *Peace and Conflict: Journal of Peace Psychology* 18, no. 3 (2012): 255, 261.

blaming others: Ibid., 259.

"interests of nation building": "Minister Michael Masutha: Parole Decision on Inmates Barnard, de Kock, and Lewis."

210 *never be forgiven:* See in particular the work of Christopher Browning, Emile Fackenheim, and Ron Rosenbaum as cited in Pumla Gobodo-Madikizela, *A Human Being Died That Night: A South African Woman Confronts the Legacy of Apartheid* (New York: First Mariner Books, 2004), 16–17.

"problem in our country": Gobodo-Madikizela, *Dare We Hope?* loc. 1544.

democratic system: Ibid., loc. 1192.

"would be a start": Ibid., loc. 280.

211 *"moral humanity?":* Ibid., loc. 300.

Afterword: Love, a Future

215 *volleyball games:* Holly Yan, Kristina Sgueglia, and Kylie Walker, "'Make America White Again': Hate Speech and Crimes Post-Election," CNN.com, December 22, 2016, http://www.cnn.com/2016/11/10/us/post-election-hate-crimes-and-fears-trnd/.

black families: Josh Feldman, "Hillary: White People Need to 'Start Listening to Legitimate Cries' About Police Shootings," *Mediaite,* July 8, 2016, http://www.mediaite.com/tv/hillary-white-people-need to-start-listening-to-legitimate-cries-about-police-shootings/.

conjure more empathy: Jonathan Lloyd, "LAPD Chief Calls for 'Empathy' at Somber LAPD Graduation Ceremony," NBC Southern California, July 8, 2016, http://www.nbclosangeles.com/news/local/Dallas-Sniper-Attacks-LAPD-Police-Officer-Shootings-386006831.html.

Syrians surviving it: James Delahoussaye, "Virtual Games Try to Generate Real Empathy for Faraway Conflict," NPR, January 25, 2015, http://www.npr.org/sections/alltechconsidered/2015/01/25/379417927/virtual-games-try-to-generate-real-empathy-for-faraway-conflict.

216 *"an empathic drive":* These quotes come from Jeremy Rifkin's TED Talk on his book *The Empathic Civilization: The Race to Global Consciousness in a World in Crisis* (New York: TarcherPerigee, 2009), https://www.ted.com/talks/jeremy_rifkin_on_the_empathic_civilization.
newly expanded identity: Ibid.

217 *natural order:* Luc Ferry, *On Love: A Philosophy for the Twenty-First Century,* transl. Andrew Brown (Cambridge: Polity Press, 2013), 12, 14, 16, 26.

218 *lineage, and economics:* Ibid., 45, 48.
youth is lionized: Ibid., 119, 131.
adventure of real love: Alain Badiou, *In Praise of Love,* transl. Peter Bush (New York: New Press, 2009), 6–9.

219 *primitive instinct:* R. Allot, "Evolutionary Aspects of Love and Empathy," *Journal of Social and Evolutionary Systems* 15, no. 4 (1992): 353–370.

Index